A SURGEONS' GUIDE
TO CARDIAC DIAGNOSIS

PART I

THE DIAGNOSTIC APPROACH

BY

DONALD N. ROSS
B. Sc., M. B., CH. B., F. R. C. S.
CONSULTANT THORACIC SURGEON
GUY'S HOSPITAL, LONDON

INTRODUCTORY NOTE
BY
PROFESSOR R. ZENKER, MUNICH

WITH 86 FIGURES
5 OF THESE COLOURED

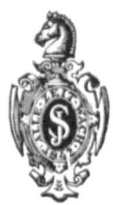

Springer-Verlag Berlin Heidelberg GmbH

1962

ISBN 978-3-540-02901-4   ISBN 978-3-642-85482-8 (eBook)
DOI 10.1007/978-3-642-85482-8

© Springer-Verlag Berlin Heidelberg 1962
Originally published by Springer-Verlag OHG Berlin · Göttingen · Heidelberg in 1962
Softcover reprint of the hardcover 1st edition 1962

Printed by J. P. Peter, Gebr. Holstein, Rothenburg o. d. Tbr.

Introductory Note*

On the occasion of a visit to Sir RUSSELL BROCK in London in 1956, and during the visit of his associate, Mr. DONALD ROSS, to Marburg in 1958, I became acquainted with the method of examination of the heart and circulation as practised by the surgeons at Guy's Hospital. Their approach was convincing because of it's simplicity and because of the wealth of information it yielded. My view was confirmed by Professor H. E. BOCK, Dr. P. SCHÖLMERICH, Dr. G. SCHETTLER and Dr. E. STEIN, the experienced cardiological members of our Marburg study group who were also impressed with the method of cardiac examination, demonstrated by Mr. DONALD N. ROSS.

The technique practised by Sir RUSSELL BROCK and his associates attempts to establish the diagnosis on the basis of careful observation and a proper interpretation of the symptoms and signs of the cardiac patient as presented to the human senses. The resulting findings are then brought into accord with the evidence obtained from the more specialised diagnostic procedures, such as x-ray examination, electrocardiography, phonocardiography, cardiac catheterisation and angiography. I believe this classical approach to cardiac diagnosis deserves more emphasis at this time of often blind reliance upon allegedly objective methods of diagnosis.

Jointly with the publishers, Springer Verlag, I am indebted to Mr. DONALD N. ROSS for complying with our request to write this introductory booklet which is modestly entitled "A Surgeons' Guide to Cardiac Diagnosis". This publication is to be followed by a second volume, dealing with indications for surgery and operative procedure in congenital and acquired cardiac disease.

I am convinced that this booklet, in it's concise and strictly scientific form, will be of interest not only to those engaged in cardiac surgery but also to the general practitioner and internist. It leads the way to simple and effective cardiac diagnosis which, due to the recent progress in surgical treatment, has gained so much in importance.

R. ZENKER, Munich

---

* Translation by Dr. H. G. BORST, Munich

Geleitwort

Anläßlich eines Besuches bei Sir Russell Brock in London im Herbst 1956 und während eines Aufenthaltes seines Schülers Donald Ross im Frühjahr 1958 in Marburg a. d. Lahn lernte ich eine Untersuchungsmethode des Herzens und des Kreislaufes kennen, die mich durch ihre Einfachheit und Folgerichtigkeit und durch die hieraus sich ergebenden Schlüsse und Entscheidungen sehr beeindruckte und überzeugte. In dieser Auffassung wurde ich durch die Zustimmung bestärkt, die das Untersuchungsvorgehen von Donald Ross bei den in der Kardiologie erfahrenen Internisten unseres Marburger Arbeitskreises, den Herren H. E. Bock, G. Schettler, P. Schölmerich und E. Stein, fand.

Das Prinzip der von Sir Russell Brock und seinen Schülern geübten Untersuchungstechnik besteht — kurz gesagt — darin, die mit den menschlichen Sinnen erfaßten und durch Überlegungen gedeuteten Symptome als wichtigste Grundlage für die Diagnostik der Herzerkrankungen zu betrachten und mit diesen Befunden, deren Feststellung jedem Arzt möglich ist, die Ergebnisse aller technischen Untersuchungsverfahren (Röntgenuntersuchung, Elektrokardiographie, Phonokardiographie, Herzkatheterismus, Angiokardiographie u. a.) in Einklang zu bringen. In einer Zeit der Überwertung angeblich objektiver Registrierverfahren ist, glaube ich, eine Erneuerung und Betonung der früheren klassischen Untersuchungen des Herzens im Rahmen der gesamten Herzdiagnostik äußerst nützlich.

Zusammen mit dem Springer-Verlag bin ich Herrn Donald Ross sehr dankbar, daß er unserer Bitte entsprochen hat, diese Einführung in die moderne Diagnostik, die bescheiden als "A Surgeons' Guide to Cardiac Diagnosis" betitelt ist, zu verfassen. Dem vorliegenden Bändchen soll ein zweites über Indikationen und Operationsverfahren der angeborenen und erworbenen Herzerkrankungen folgen.

Ich bin überzeugt, daß das Werk nicht nur die in der Herzchirurgie tätigen Chirurgen, sondern auch praktische Ärzte und Internisten interessieren wird, da es jedem ein zu neuer Bedeutung gelangtes Gebiet, die Herzdiagnostik, in knapper, aber doch streng wissenschaftlicher Form erschließt. R. Zenker, München

Preface

This book in no way purports to be a substitute for standard textbooks on cardiological diagnosis. This would be both pretentious and pointless since large sections of cardiology are at this stage, outside the scope of surgery. Also there are a number of "surgical" lesions which do not require surgical relief.

The successful management of cardiac disability requires the unterstanding and co-operation of physicians and surgeons working as a team. The surgeon, however, should not evade his responsibilities. In cardiac surgery there is a need for the same clinical assessment which he exercises every day in the treatment of so-called general surgical conditions. It is to help him in this task that this book is directed.

Acknowledgements

It is with pleasure that I acknowledge my indebteness to Sir RUSSELL BROCK under whose guiding hand I have trained as a cardiac surgeon.

More directly, I am grateful to Dr. JANE SOMERVILLE and Dr. ALAN JOHNSON, both of whom have spent long hours reading the manuscript and correcting my errors. Dr. BLÖMER of Munich has also made valuable suggestions.

Mr. F. MUIR of the Cardiac Department, Guy's Hospital, and Dr. M. LESSOF, have been helpful in collecting a number of illustrative electrocardiographs and phonocardiographs. These are the property of the Cardiac Department of Guy's Hospital and I am grateful to Dr. CHARLES BAKER and Dr. DENNIS DEUCHAR for permission to reproduce them.

Dr. JOHN DOW of the Department of Diagnostic Radiology has supplied the radiographs and Mr. JOHN GAZET, F.R.C.S. took the photographs, while my house surgeon Mr. B. A. ROSS acted as a photographic model.

I am particularly grateful to the publishers for the patience in dealing with the problems arising from distance, postal delays and language differences.

London   D. N. R.

Contents

CHAPTER I

Introduction

In spite of the rapid development of cardiac surgery over the past ten years and the complexity of modern cardiological diagnostic techniques, clinical assessment remains the foundation on which treatment must be based.

In order to develop sound clinical judgement, it is the responsibility of the cardiac surgeon to familiarise himself with the tools of bedside and laboratory diagnosis of heart disease. He can then make full use of his unique opportunities for studying the living heart. At operation, he can note the effects of the haemodynamic burden imposed by the disease process. Daily he is confronted with visual evidence of the effects of these burdens and, by inspection and palpation of the heart and the use of electromanometry, he is able to confirm the preoperative diagnosis to a degree of accuracy denied to his physician colleagues and to the pathologist in the autopsy room.

Cardiology is a wide field and embraces many conditions outside the present and probable future scope of surgery; but the surgically important conditions fall largely within a field familiar to all generally trained surgeons. To these, well-tried general surgical principles can be applied. Surgeons are familiar with the diagnosis and treatment of obstruction to hollow muscular organs including the gut, urinary and biliary tract. The heart and vascular tree can, in this respect, be regarded as a highly developed hollow muscular system which propels blood instead of chyme or bile and is subject to the same burdens of obstruction, malfunction or incompetence and internal fistulae. Obstructed and regurgitant valves and communications between the systemic and pulmonary circuits constitute the great majority of surgically correctable cardiovascular deformities.

We have to regard the cardiovascular system in terms of two simple but highly-efficient pumps and we must familiarise ourselves with the evidence of any departure from their normal working.

The major vessels entering and leaving the heart are less specialised extensions of the muscular cardiac tube, but should be regarded as part of the cardiovascular tree. They are subject to the same general disease processes and are susceptible to similar diagnostic methods and treatment.

Historical Background

The earliest attempts at cardiac surgery were largely related to the management of trauma, pericardial tamponade, and the removal of foreign bodies. A notable landmark was the first mitral valvotomy performed by SOUTTAR in 1925, by a technique identical with that used in countless hospitals throughout the world today. Cardiological opinion was not ready to accept this advance, being preoccupied at that time with the importance of the myocardium in this condition.

It was not until 1939 when GROSS first successfully ligated a persistent ductus arteriosus that cardiac surgery took its place among the major surgical specialities. This event was followed in 1945 by the treatment of an aortic coarctation (CRAFOORD and GROSS) and, in the same year, the BLALOCK-TAUSSIG operation for cyanotic congenital heart disease was described. Although these operations are included in the term "cardiac surgery" they are, technically, operations upon the great vessels. The present era of surgery upon the heart itself was introduced by SELLORS and BROCK in 1948 in relation to stenosis of the pulmonary valve, and at about the same time, BAILEY, BROCK and HARKEN all reported the successful re-introduction of Souttar's operation for mitral stenosis.

Further advances have been rapid. Obstructive lesions of all four heart valves are now regularly treated and the introduction of hypothermia by BIGELOW in 1952 paved the way for successful closure of atrial septal defects under vision.

Work on the heart-lung apparatus, pioneered by GIBBON of Philadelphia, has resulted in the introduction of a number of successful machines, which have opened up a new field of deliberate, unhurried intra-cardiac surgery. The closure of ventricular septal defects is now commonplace, and a wide variety of lesions has become amenable to surgery.

At present, efforts are being directed towards the surgical treatment of coronary insufficiency, and valve regurgitation remains a problem of importance. A possible solution of this latter condition lies in achieving successful valve replacement with prostheses or homografts, but tissue grafts are subject to the well recognised difficulties of tissue incompatibility.

Total cardiac transplantation has been achieved technically on a number of occasions in experimental animals. The possibility of replacing a diseased heart awaits a solution of the immunological problem.

The related field of blood vessel surgery has kept pace with these advances, and the treatment of aneurysms and obstructive lessions of the aorta and major blood vessels is common surgical practice.

CHAPTER II

Anatomical Considerations

A sound anatomical knowledge is one of the pillars upon which accurate diagnosis must rest. The gross anatomy of the heart and its relationship to the lungs and other intrathoracic structures, while of fundamental importance, is outside the scope of this work. Only those features having a particular bearing on cardiac surgery will be mentioned. One point worth emphasizing is that the living anatomy of the heart as observed by the surgeon, often bears little resemblance to the formalin-hardened post-mortem specimens seen in museums or as illustrations in textbooks of anatomy.

Some knowledge of the embryology of the heart is essential to a clear understanding of the cardiac septa and of the various congenital cardiac malformations.

Embryology

The heart is developed from a simple muscular tube which collects blood at one end (sinus venosus) and discharges it at the other end (truncus arteriosus) into the branchial arches.

Very early in its development the cardiac tube differentiates into five separate portions — sinus venosus, common atrium, common ventricle, bulbus cordis, and truncus arteriosus. From this stage, the tube, growing within the confines of the pericardium and fixed at each end, flexes acutely upon itself in the region between the ventricle and the bulbus cordis. At about this time, the sinus venosus fuses progressively into the common atrium. Where the walls of the ventricle and the bulbus cordis are in apposition, they form the bulbo-ventricular septum which becomes largely absorbed in the subsequent development of the heart.

At this early stage, one recognises the atrio-ventricular junction or atrio-ventricular canal (p. 6), which will be the site of the atrio-ventricular valves

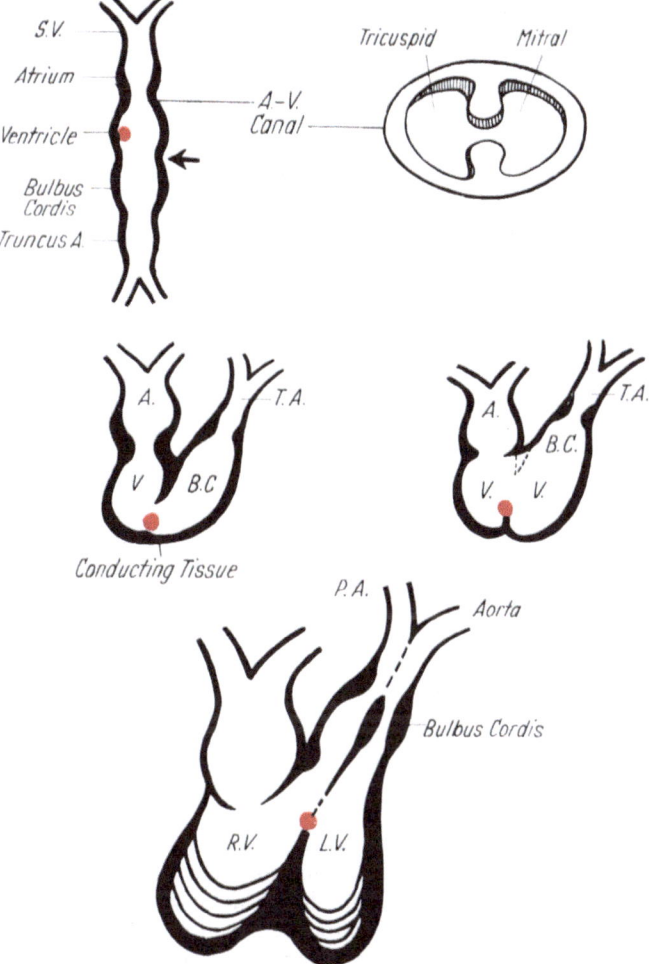

Fig. 1. Stages in the development of the heart from a simple tube

(tricuspid and mitral). Also the common ventricle now presents an inflow portion and outflow portion, the latter being derived from the bulbus cordis. This pattern is retained in the fully developed heart.

Elements of the bulbus cordis contribute to the outflow tract of both right and left ventricles. In addition it will be seen that an area of the ventricular wall contains the specialised cardiac muscle which later forms the conducting tissue or bundle of His. As far as the true ventricles are concerned, their subsequent development is dependent upon the formation of the ventricular septum.

The right and left ventricular cavities are formed as hollowings-out or evaginations of the thick spongy muscular wall, leaving a muscular ridge between them. Along the free margin of this ridge is located the conducting tissue.

At the same time two ridges develop within the bulbus cordis dividing it into right and left ventricular outflow portions. These ridges grow down towards the rudimentory ventricular septum and complete the separation of the two ventricles.

There is a deficiency where the muscular components of the ventricular septum meet and this is bound inferiorly by the conducting tissue. This defect is filled in by endocardial proliferation and constitutes the membranous part of the ventricular septum.

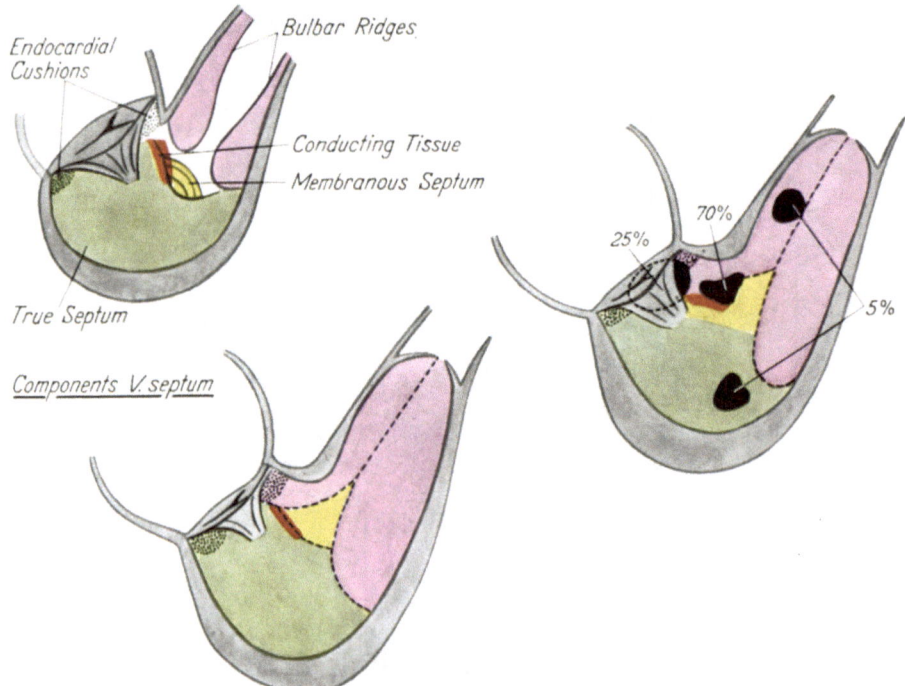

Fig. 2. The development of the ventricular septum showing the location of the common ventricular septal defects

It may now be appreciated that the common ventricular septal defects are likely to occur in the region of the membranous part of the septum where the various components come together. Further, the intimate relation of the conduction bundle to the lower (postero-inferior) margin of the defect is explained.

The atrial septum has an equally complex embryological development — the complexity being dictated by the need for maintaining an uninterrupted right-to-left shunt of oxygenated blood from the placenta throughout foetal life.

The first subdivision of the common atrial chamber is by the septum primum which grows down from the vault of the atrium and has a crescentic deficiency, or ostium primum, inferiorly. This ostium primum lies immediately above the forming atrio-ventricular valves. Failure of the septum to unite with the endocardial cushions of the atrio-ventricular canal can result in the ostium primum type of atrial septal defect or any variation of the atrio-ventricular canal deformity.

A thicker septum secundum grows down on the right side of the septum primum, extending downwards and forwards to cover the crescentic ostium primum. This septum is deficient posteriorly — the floor of the deficiency being formed by the thin septum primum and the whole saucer-like area being called the fossa ovalis.

A hole now appears higher in the septum primum. This is the ostium secundum and with the fossa ovalis deficiency in the septum secundum forms a one-way flap valve. This is the foramen ovale, which persists in adult life in about 30 per cent of people.

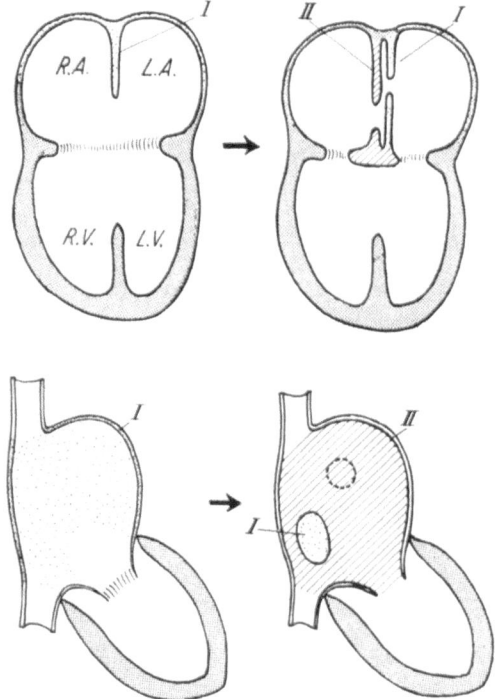

Fig. 3. The development of the atrial septum as seen diagrammatically in antero-posterior and lateral projection. I. septum primum. II. septum secundum

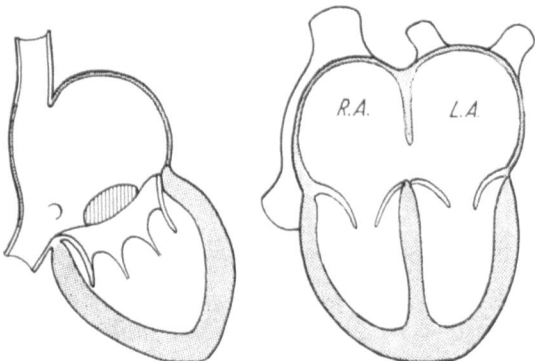

Fig. 4. The ostium primum defect lateral and antero-posterior views

Any breakdown or failure of development of the septum primum in the floor of the fossa ovalis leaves a large defect posteriorly in the atrial septum and is the common type of atrial septal defect encountered. It is commonly called the ostium secundum defect to distinguish it from the ostium primum type, but is more accurately a fossa ovalis type of defect.

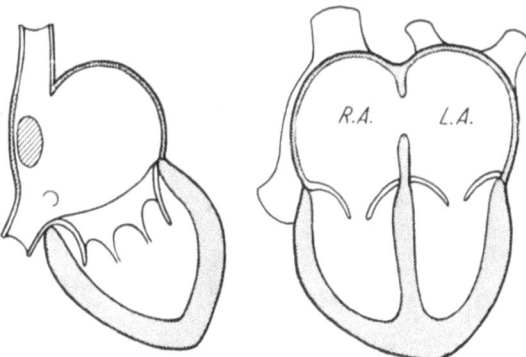

Fig. 5. The ostium secundum defect as seen in lateral and antero-posterior projection

The Atrio-Ventricular Canal

That part of the primitive cardiac tube between the common atrium and the common ventricle is known as the atrio-ventricular canal. In this area, dorsal and ventral endocardial cushions protrude and join to divide the canal into mitral and tricuspid orifices with their corresponding valves. Above, these cushions fuse with the atrial septum, and below with the ventricular septum.

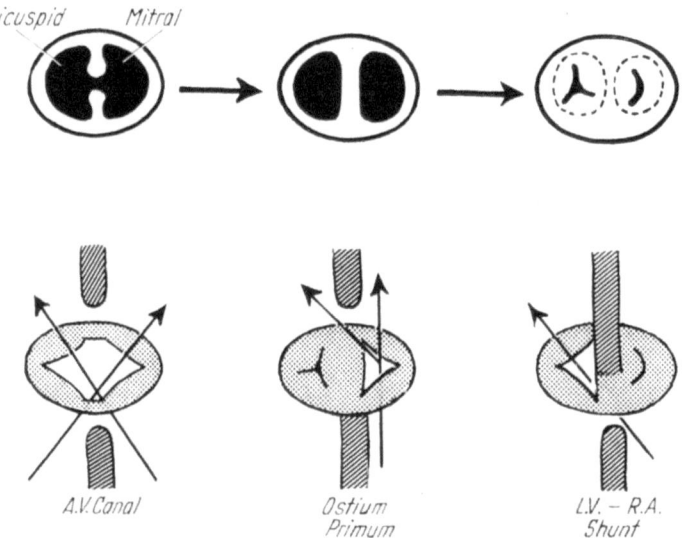

Fig. 6. The development of the atrio-ventricular canal and the possible defects resulting from incomplete fusion of the endocardial cushions and the cardiac septa

Where there is an abnormality of development before the valves have formed, the condition of persistent atrio-ventricularis communis, or one of its variations like the ostium primum type of atrial septal defect results. Due to imperfect fusion of the endocardial cushion tissues there are usually associated clefts in the mitral and tricuspid valve leaflets.

The Bulbus Cordis

The interior of the ventricles can be separated into inflow and outflow portions. The former is derived from the common ventricle and the latter from the bulbus cordis. A maldevelopment of the right ventricular part of the bulbus cordis is probably responsible for the various forms of pulmonary stenosis and also the infundibular stenosis and associated ventricular septal defect characteristic of FALLOT's tetralogy.

It has been noted earlier (p. 4) that the developing bulbar ridges divide the bulbus cordis into two, the greater part forming the outflow tract of the right ventricle. The contribution of the bulbus to the left ventricular outflow tract is recognisable in the fully developed heart as the smooth-walled vestibule. The vestibule of the left ventricle lies immediately below the aortic valves, and malformations in this area are again likely to be responsible for the conditions of congenital aortic valve or subvalvar stenosis, corresponding with similar conditions in the outflow portion of the right ventricle.

The Branchial Arches

These are remnants of the gill-clefts seen in fish and each contains a vascular arch running between the ventral and dorsal aortae. The ventral aortae are connected proximally to the truncus arteriosus. The adult vascular pattern emerges

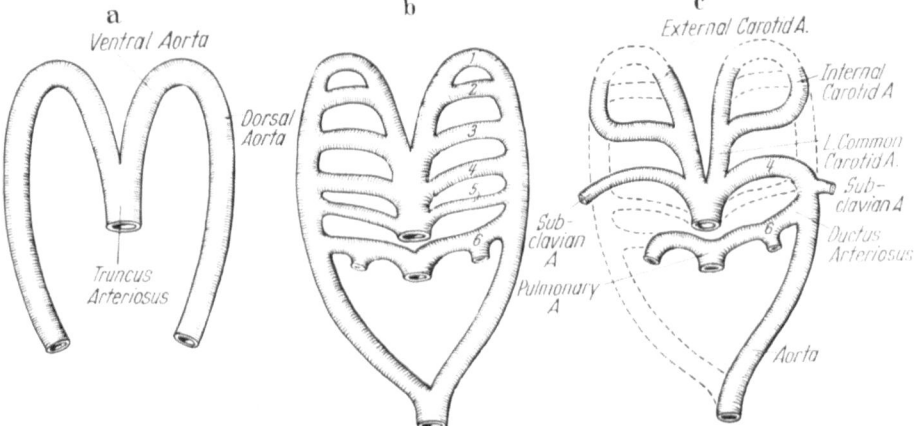

Fig. 7. The branchial arches and the development of the great vessels

as a result of absorption of most of these arches while others persist in part or wholly.

Reference to the diagram indicates that the persistence of the left fourth arch gives rise to the arch of the aorta while the 6th arch persists medially as the pulmonary artery. The connection between the lateral portion of the sixth arch and the aorta forms the ductus arteriosus which normally closes soon after birth. Persistence of the right ventral aorta or both ventral aortae results in a right aortic arch or double aortic arch. Abnormalities of the branchial arches are also responsible for coarctation of the aorta.

With regard to the anatomy of the normally developed heart, this is well described in standard textbooks.

The inclination of the septa, particularly of the atrial septum, is not generally appreciated. The atrial septum is by no means vertical and is, in fact, at a considerable angle to the vertical plane.

This fact has been used to advantage in the surgical approach to the left atrium and atrial septum (BROCK). The left atrium and mitral valve are surprisingly accessible from the right chest for the same reason, and this has led BAILEY to

advocate mitral valvotomy through the right chest. Also, open surgery of the
mitral valve is often carried out through the large protrusion of the left atrium
into the right chest. Conversely, the atrial septum is less accessible from the left side.

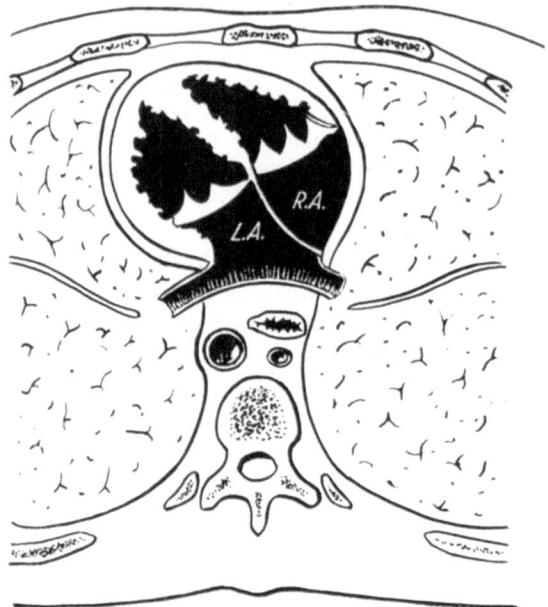

Fig. 8. A cross section of the heart showing the inclination of the atrial and ventricular septa in relation
to the chest

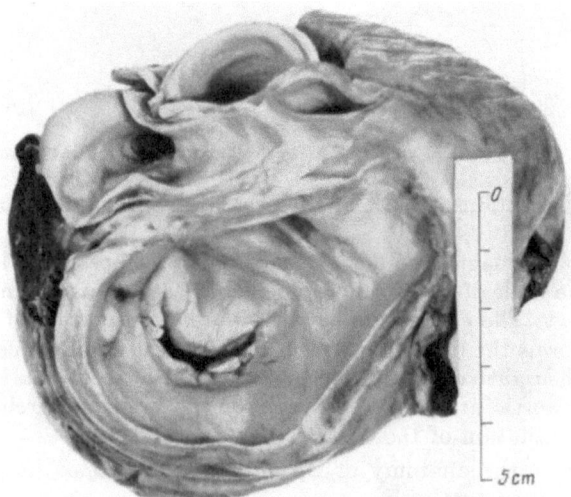

Fig. 9. Photograph of a mitral valve showing the curved orifice

The inclination of the ventricular septum has some bearing on the line of the
mitral valve orifice. The surgical anatomy of this valve has been carefully described
by BROCK but the concave fish mouth-like inclination of the valve commissures
is not always appreciated, particularly in relation to the use of cutting valvotomes.

If this fact is not born in mind, extension of the valve split in the line of the original dilatation is likely to encroach on the postero-lateral cusp resulting in regurgitation.

Elementary Haemodynamics

The maintenance of the pulmonary and systemic circulations is dependent upon the output of the ventricles and the resistances they encounter. The result of the ventricles discharging their blood into narrowing tubes is to cause the pressure of the blood in these tubes to rise to the point at which the resistance to forward flow is overcome. The blood pressure is, therefore, a measure of the cardiac output and the peripheral resistance.

$$B.P. = C.O. \times P.R.$$

In the normal state the output of the right and left ventricles is identical, yet the mean blood pressure recorded in the pulmonary artery is only about 20 mm. Hg

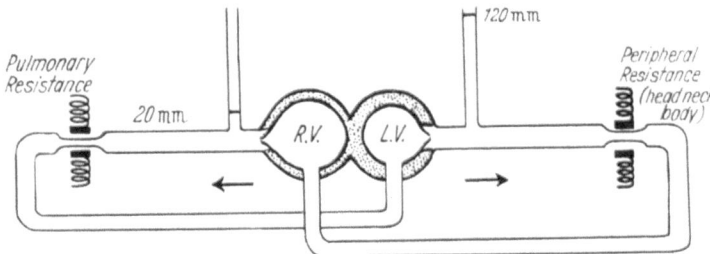

Fig. 10. The high pressure generated in the systemic bed is the result of the high peripheral resistance

while that in the aorta is about 100 mm. Hg. Therefore, it can be inferred that the peripheral obstruction (or resistance) met with in the systemic vascular bed is much greater than that of the pulmonary vascular bed.

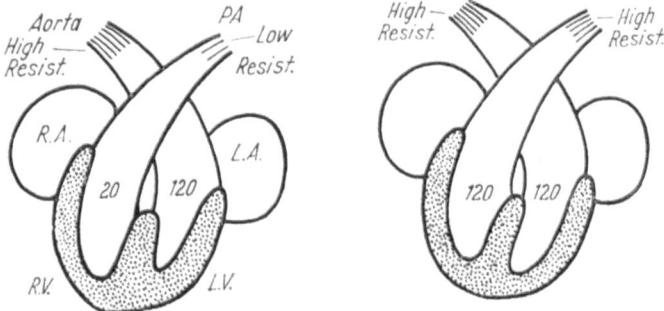

Fig. 11. Where the resistance offered by the lung vessels approaches to that of the peripheral vessels, the pressure in the right ventricle rises — pulmonary hypertension

Just as one can have factors which increase the systemic vascular resistance and give rise to a high blood pressure, so one can have changes in the pulmonary vessels which increase the peripheral resistance in the lungs. Consequently the pulmonary artery pressure rises. This explains one type of pulmonary hypertension or, more accurately, pulmonary hypertension secondary to increased pulmonary resistance.

Pulmonary Hypertension

This term tends to be used loosely and without an adequate understanding of the underlying mechanisms. It simply means a raised pulmonary artery pressure

above the normally accepted systolic value of 20—30 mm. Hg. There are a number
of possible causes which can be classified as follows:

Primary Pulmonary Hypertension
Secondary Pulmonary Hypertension $\left\{\begin{array}{l}\text{Passive}\\\text{Active}\end{array}\right.$ $\left\{\begin{array}{l}\text{Secondary to increased flow}\\\text{Secondary to increased resistance}\end{array}\right.$

Most cases of "surgical" pulmonary hypertension are secondary to some underlying cardiac malformation or disease. So-called primary pulmonary hypertension
arises with no obvious cause and there are well marked changes in the peripheral

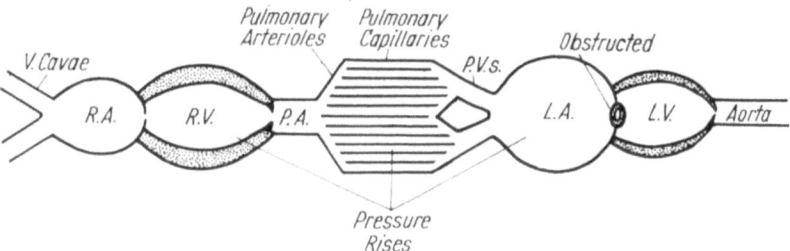

Fig. 12. With the two sides of the heart and the lungs represented as a single tube, it is seen that the
pressure rises in that part of the circulation intervening between the obstructed valve and the active
right ventricle

lung vascularity as in systemic hypertension. Some of these changes are un-
doubtedly the result of generalised lung disease and there is good evidence in
support if the theory that multiple pulmonary emboli with blocking of the peripheral vessels is another probable cause.

Secondary pulmonary hypertension is of more concern to cardiac surgeons,
particularly in relation to intracardiac shunts.

Passive pulmonary hypertension is easily understood and commonly results
from obstruction at the mitral orifice or from left ventricular failure. The right
ventricle continues to pump blood into the lung vessels and the pressure within
them rises to a level at which the obstruction is overcome or until the left heart
can deal with the load (fig. 12).

Active pulmonary hypertension arises either as a result of increased pulmonary
blood flow or because of increased resistance in the pulmonary vascular bed, or
a combination of these.

The increased pulmonary artery pressure arising from increased *flow* is also
known as hyperdynamic pulmonary hypertension. Reduction of the flow to physiological levels by closure of a septal defect results in restoration of the pulmonary artery pressure to normal. It should be noted that these cases have a normal
pulmonary vascular resistance, the rise in pressure being purely a flow phenomenon.

Some cases of left-to-right shunt, particularly those due to ventricular septal
defect and, to a lesser extent, with persistent ductus arteriosus, not only have an
increased flow giving rise to a raised pulmonary artery pressure, but there are often
associated changes in the peripheral lung vessels. These changes actively increase
the pulmonary vascular resistance and it is important to evaluate this factor
since correction of the shunt in these cases will not always restore the pulmonary
artery pressure to normal.

In some instances the raised resistance acts as a gross obstruction and if there
is a septal defect present, desaturated right heart blood escapes into the left heart
chambers causing cyanosis. This is the mechanism of the cyanosis in the Eisen-

menger group of conditions. In these, the septal defect plays the part of a safety valve for the right ventricle and closure of the defect is contraindicated until such time that means of reducing the pulmonary vascular resistance may be developed.

The cause of the increased pulmonary vascular resistance in ventricular septal defect and some cases of ductus is a matter for speculation. Also the rarity of this phenomenon in uncomplicated atrial septal defect is of interest. Where an increased pulmonary resistance is encountered in atrial septal defect in the younger age group, it is sufficiently rare to make one suspect an incorrect diagnosis or a complicated type of atrial defect. However at a later age in atrial septal defect or, indeed, with any type of left-to-right shunt, thrombosis in the dilated pulmonary vessels is quite common and is then a cause of the terminal rise of pulmonary artery pressure and cyanosis from reversal of the shunt.

A high pulmonary artery resistance is common in young patients with a ventricular septal defect. Where the defect is large, an increased pulmonary vascular resistance approaching that in the systemic vascular bed prevents flooding of the lungs with blood from the left ventricle.

The most widely accepted explanation for the increased pulmonary vascular resistance in ventricular septal defect is that it represents a persistence into adult

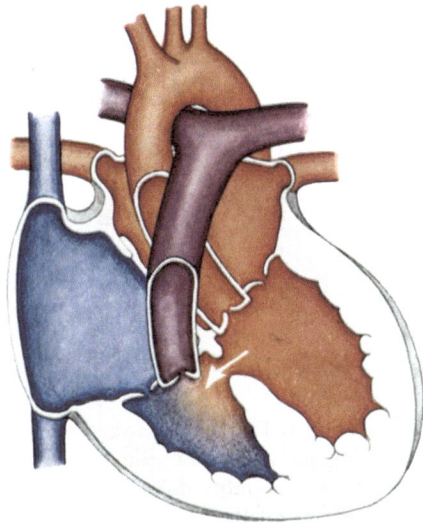

Fig. 13. This shows the course of the blood from both right and left ventricles into the pulmonary artery which represents a path of reduced resistance in a straight forword case of ventricular septal defect

life of the high resistance and blood vessel pattern found in the foetus. Histological studies bear this out in that there is a close similarity between the pulmonary vasculature in ventricular septal defect and in foetal lung tissue.

Before birth the lungs are functionless and the resistance offered to blood flow by the tortuous and muscular pulmonary arteries and arterioles in the airless lungs is very considerably greater than that of the systemic vascular resistance.

At birth the lungs become aerated and with expansion, the tortuous pulmonary vessels straighten out. This reduces their resistance to a level corresponding with that of the systemic vascular bed (WOOD, 1958).

In normal circumstances the pulmonary vascular resistance then regresses slowly during the succeeding early months of life. The muscular arterioles thin out and approach the adult pattern and, with this, the pulmonary resistance and the pulmonary artery pressure falls to adult levels. This sequence of events can be followed histologically and lung biopsy at operation can be of help in assessing the degree of pulmonary vascular resistance. Also, the electrocardiogram reflects the changing resistance in that it shows a dominance of the right ventricle at birth and as the pulmonary resistance falls the electrocardiogram approaches that of the adult type with an increasing left ventricular dominance. The cause of this regression of the pulmonary vascular resistance and the accompanying change from muscular to elastic type of thin-walled arteries is not known.

Where the child is born with a ventricular septal defect, the initial fall of pulmonary resistance probably occurs when the child breathes and expands the lung vessels. However, as far as we are aware, the subsequent changes in the muscular arteries and the accompanying fall of pulmonary artery pressure does not progress as in the uncomplicated case. If there is no fall in pulmonary resistance, pulmonary and aortic pressures are equal and no shunt occurs across the ventricular

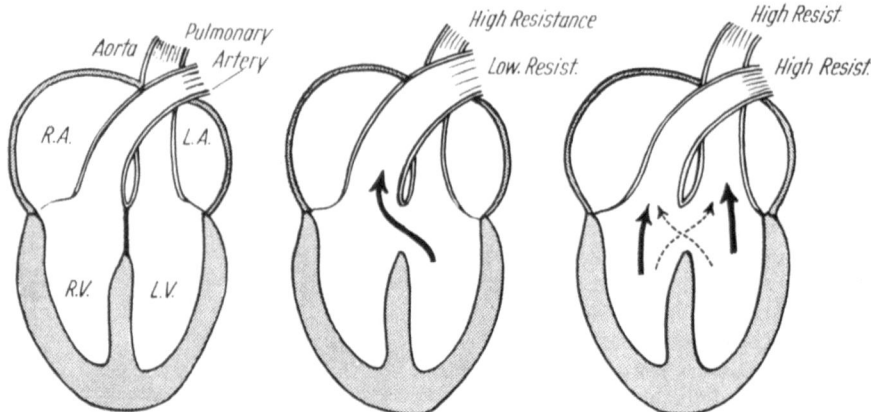

Fig. 14. This shows the effect of the pulmonary resistance on the blood flow across a ventricular septal defect. With a low resistance, the shunt is predominantly left-to-right and with a high resistance, it is balanced

septal defect. In fact, temporary elevations of pulmonary artery resistance with straining and crying are likely to reverse the shunt and produce cyanosis.

Where the pulmonary resistance starts to regress, the left ventricle will discharge some of its contents via the ventricular septal defect into the pulmonary

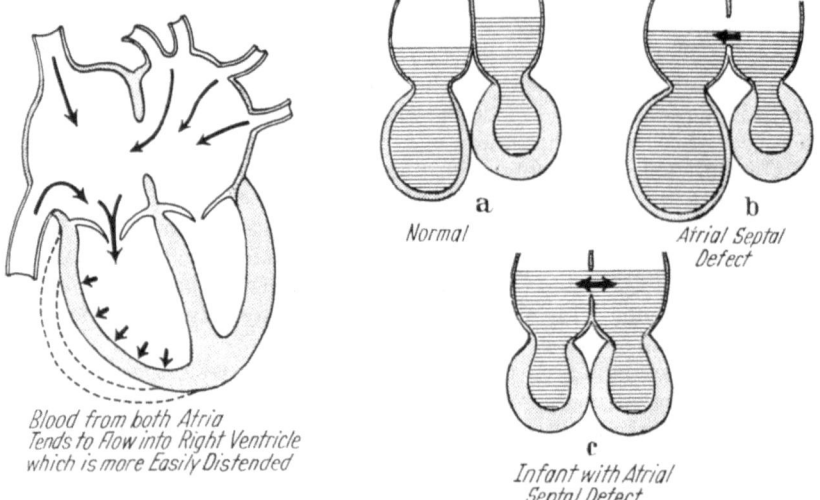

Fig. 15. The flow of blood in atrial septal defect is in the direction of the more distensible ventricle during diastole. In the infant with atrial septal defect (c) both ventricles are equally muscular so that flow across the defect is minimal

artery, which represents a path of reduced resistance. Should the pulmonary resistance continue to fall, progressively more blood will shunt across the ventricular septal defect into the lung bed, giving rise to the full clinical picture of ventricular septal defect with a heavy left-to-right shunt (fig. 13).

At some point the fall of pulmonary resistance must be opposed, otherwise all the left ventricular blood would be discharged into the pulmonary artery and none would pass into the aorta — a condition incompatible with life. In other words, the increased pulmonary resistance serves to counter an excessive discharge of left ventricular blood into the lungs. This is the usual picture in cases of ventricular septal defect surviving the first months of life. There is an elevation of pulmonary artery pressure with an element of muscular hypertrophy of the lung vessels and a persistence of some right ventricular hypertrophy in the electro-cardiograph as evidence of the raised pulmonary resistance.

A similar explanation can account for the finding of an increased pulmonary resistance in cases of large ductus arteriosus where the raised resistance in the peripheral lung fields again limits a catastrophic shunt of blood across the ductus.

It has been noted clinically and at cardiac catheterization that a raised pulmonary resistance and pulmonary artery pressure are uncommon in cases of atrial septal defect. An acceptable explanation for this observation has been offered by WOOD (1958). He proposes that in atrial septal defect the normal regression of the pulmonary resistance can take place, since there is probably no shunt occurring at birth. The pulmonary artery resistance falls progressively to a normal level and there is an accompanying steady resolution of the right ventricular hypertrophy. It is only when the right ventricle has thinned and become more distensible that a shunt of blood across the atrial septal defect becomes significant. By that time the pulmonary resistance and right ventricular pressure are probably normal. Any rise of pulmonary artery pressure now is simply due to an increased flow (hyperdynamic pulmonary hypertension) or later as a result of thrombosis in the pulmonary vessels.

Post-Stenotic Dilatation

Dilatation of the vessels or chambers of the heart occurs beyond an obstruction and is particularly noticeable on chest radiography or at operation. Thus, one sees post-stenotic dilatation of the main pulmonary artery trunk in cases of pulmonary valve stenosis or a similar dilatation of the ascending aorta in aortic valve stenosis. Post-stenotic dilatations also occur beyond obstructions in other parts of the vascular tree and within the heart chambers. An important illustration of this latter feature is the post-stenotic thin-walled infundibular chamber seen in cases of pulmonary infundibular stenosis. This has been described by BROCK and is characteristic of many cases of FALLOT's tetralogy with infundibular stenosis.

The exact mechanism of post-stenotic dilatation has not been settled conclusively but HOLMAN has made a great contribution to the understanding of the condition by showing that it is a physical phenomenon not peculiar to the human vascular system. He demonstrated simply and convincingly in his laboratory that an ordinary rubber tube, when connected with a source of flowing water would develop a post-stenotic bulge beyond a point of constriction.

This may be in some way related to fatigue of the rubber structure but also indicates that there are considerable lateral forces in operation beyond the obstruction. Also, turbulence beyond the obstruction may have the effect of distending the vessel wall in this region.

Pressure Relationships in the Cardiovascular System

It has been mentioned (p. 9) that the aortic and pulmonary artery pressures are normally in the ratio of about six to one, as a result of the unequal resistance in the pulmonary and systemic vascular beds.

If the cardiovascular system is again considered as a tubular pump (as it developed embryologically), the circulation can be represented quite simply.

The pressure in the right ventricle generally varies between 20—30/0 in systole and diastole, and that in the left ventricle is about 120/0. If there is no obstruction at the pulmonary or aortic valve, the systolic pressure will be transmitted unaltered from the ventricles to the main vessels. As the pressure falls towards zero

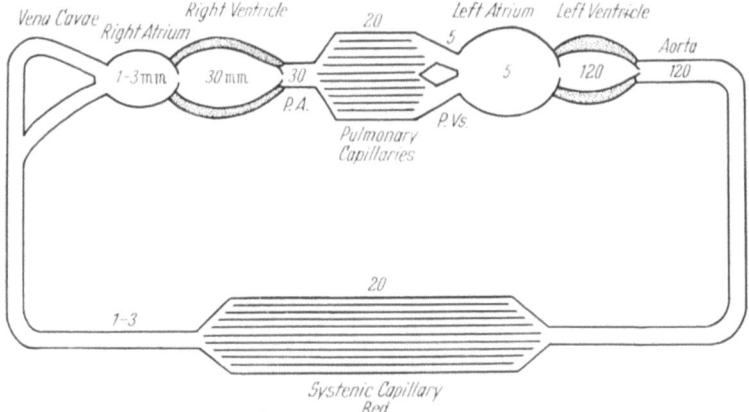

Fig. 16. Figure to illustrate the pressure relationship within the cardiovascular system

in the ventricles the pulmonary and aortic valves close. This is the mechanism which maintains the diastolic pressure and a continuous forward flow throughout the cardiac cycle. Thus, in the pulmonary artery the pressures are 20—30/5—15 mm. and in the aorta about 120/80 mm.

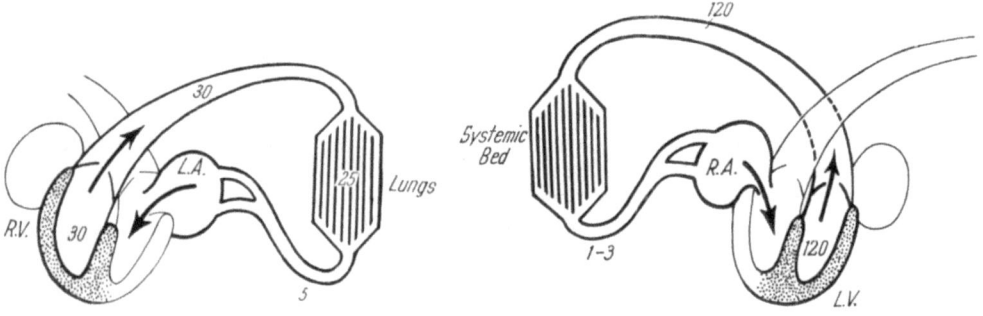

Fig. 17   Fig. 18

Fig. 17. The right ventricle is responsible for driving the blood through the lungs, the left atrium and the mitral valve. Left atrial contraction contributes little to the forward flow

Fig. 18. The left ventricle drives the blood through the systemic bed, great veins and the right atrium

As the blood ejected from the right ventricle flows through the rapidly dividing and narrowing pulmonary circulation, its pressure falls and is about 5—10 mm. by the time it reaches the pulmonary veins and left atrium. The normal mean pressure in the left atrium is, therefore, about 5—10 mm. and this pressure is generated by the *right* ventricle. This fundamental fact is often overlooked. Conseqently when the outflow of the left atrium (mitral valve) is obstructed, the right ventricle continues to push blood into the lungs and left atrium at increased pressure in order to overcome the obstruction. This results in a rise of pulmonary artery pressure (passive pulmonary hypertension, p. 10) and congested lungs. The symptoms of cough, dyspnoea, and haemoptysis are a result of this congestion. If the pressure in the lung capillaries rises above the plasma osmotic pressure and ability of the lymphatics to deal with the excess transudation of fluid, pulmonary oedema results. These features are not the result of a failing heart but arise because of *increased* efforts on the part of the right ventricle.

Similarly, the left ventricle provides the drive and pressure to force blood through the systemic vascular bed and venae cavae into the right atrium. Where there is obstruction at the tricuspid valve or where the right ventricle is unable to cope with its burden, the left ventricle continues to force blood on, and there is a rise of pressure in the systemic venous bed. There is consequently a raised venous pressure and peripheral oedema; exactly analagous with the raised pressure in the pulmonary bed and pulmonary oedema.

The Venous Return

It has been pointed out that the continuous flow of blood through the great veins into the right atrium is largely the result of the left ventricular propulsive force. This fact is often obscured when undue attention is paid to the other factors modifying and influencing the venous return.

Table. *Factors responsible for the Venous Return*

1. *The left Ventricle*
2. Other contributory factors —
    a) Leg muscles plus venous valves
    b) Negative thoracic pressure
    c) ? Contractions of veins

Muscular contractions, particularly in the legs during exercise, are a powerful *aid* to venous return, particularly in the erect position when gravity must be overcome. The valves in the veins ensure a unidirectional flow. This mechanism however, is an ancillary one and not essential, as can be demonstrated in the recumbent patient under the influence of a muscle relaxant, with abolition of all muscle tone and contraction. Venous return remains efficient.

A further factor aiding venous return is the negative pressure within the thoracic cage. This also modifies the pressure in the great veins and right atrium, but the negative pressure is not an essential factor. This fact is evident in the patient under anaesthesia with both pleural spaces open and with intermittent positive pressure respiration supplied by the anaesthetist. Again, the venous return is maintained.

A minor factor influencing venous return may be the contraction of the great veins which can be noted within the thoracic cage but this cannot contribute greatly in the absence of venous valves nearer the heart.

Effects of Obstruction and Regurgitation in the Cardiovascular System

Obstruction at the mitral and tricuspid valves has been considered. In each case the right and left ventricle respectively must pump harder in order to overcome the increased resistance and to maintain normal flow. The intervening pulmonary or systemic capillary pressure rises, and pulmonary or systemic oedema results if this rise is sufficiently high. This is the picture of *atrial* obstruction.

Where the outflow from the right or left *ventricle* is obstructed as in pulmonary or aortic stenosis, the obstructed ventricle continues to eject its blood at a higher head of pressure in order to maintain the peripheral blood flow and pressure as near normal as possible. Thus, the left ventricle may have to generate a pressure of 200—300 mm. Hg. and the right ventricle 100—200 mm. Hg. to maintain normal flow and pressure relationships in the aorta and pulmonary artery. Unfortunately, unlike atrial obstruction, no capillary bed intervenes in cases of obstruction to the ventricles so that the increased burden is carried for a long period without symptoms. During this asymptomatic period, the muscle of the affected ventricle undergoes massive concentric hypertrophy. This progressive increase of wall thickness steadily encroaches upon the lumen of the ventricular cavity.

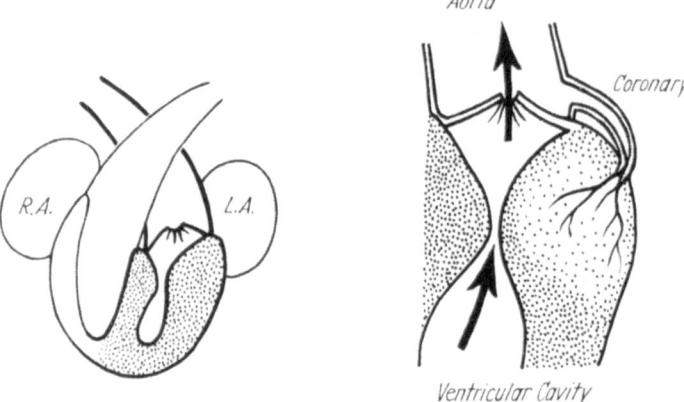

Fig. 19. The vicious circle of ventricular obstruction. Enlarged view shows how the hypertrophied muscle itself acts as an obstruction and has a deficient blood supply.

At the same time, the blood requirement of this hypertrophied muscle mass is increased. Coronary blood flow, however is probably reduced because of the prolonged systolic ejection phase during which the coronary vessels are compressed. In addition, the diminished cavity of the ventricle means that there is less filling in diastole and, consequently, less ejection with each systole to meet the increasing coronary blood requirements. As the effective stroke volume of ejected blood falls, the heart can only compensate by beating faster. This is again at the expense of the diastolic filling phase of the ventricle and the period of coronary forward flow.

In addition to this vicious circle of an increasing burden with diminishing blood supply, actual muscular obstruction to the outflow of blood can supervene as a result of hypertrophy of the ventricular outflow tract. This secondary muscular obstruction has been described by BROCK and has been demonstrated repeatedly at operation and at right and left heart catheterization. The condition and its anatomical significance can also be demonstrated in plastic casts of the ventricular cavities.

The condition of secondary muscular obstruction is most commonly recognised in the right ventricle in cases of pulmonary valve stenosis but it is also a factor of importance in left ventricular obstruction. In the presence of an hypertrophied muscular outflow, the obstruction now comes to lie proximal to the original valve stenosis, and the condition may become quite inoperable or, in certain circumstances may require resection of the hypertrophied outflow muscle.

Failure of the doubly-obstructed, hypertrophied and blood-starved ventricle is usually sudden and devastating, and this is a clinical phenomenon best recognised in cases of untreated aortic stenosis.

An awareness of the consequences of unrelieved obstruction of the ventricles emphasises the need for early relief of the obstruction before the vicious circle is established. Symptoms do not, as a rule, develop until the condition is advanced.

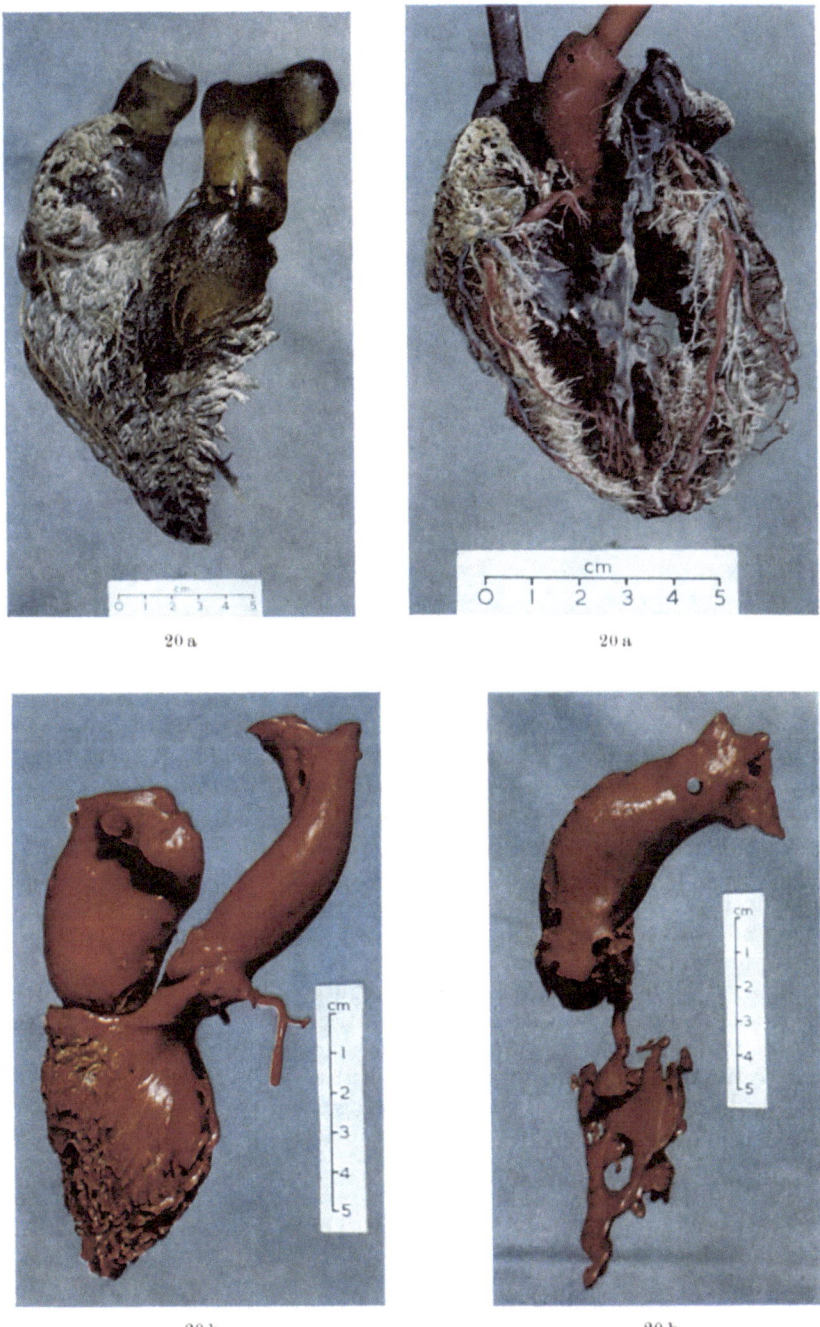

Fig. 20. Coloured plastic casts of the right and left ventricular outflow tracts

a) Shows a normal right atrium ventricle and pulmonary artery and a cast from a case of severe right ventricular obstruction showing the slit-like cavity and outflow tract

b) A normal left ventricular outflow and the result of severe aortic stenosis. A flattened left ventricular cavity leads to a lunge aorta via a thread-like outflow tract

In addition, the hypertrophy is concentric, so that one does not as a rule find a large heart on X-ray examination, even in the presence of gross obstruction, until cardiac failure occurs. The diagnosis of ventricular obstruction should be clinical, assisted by cardiac catheterization or left ventricular puncture and, if an important

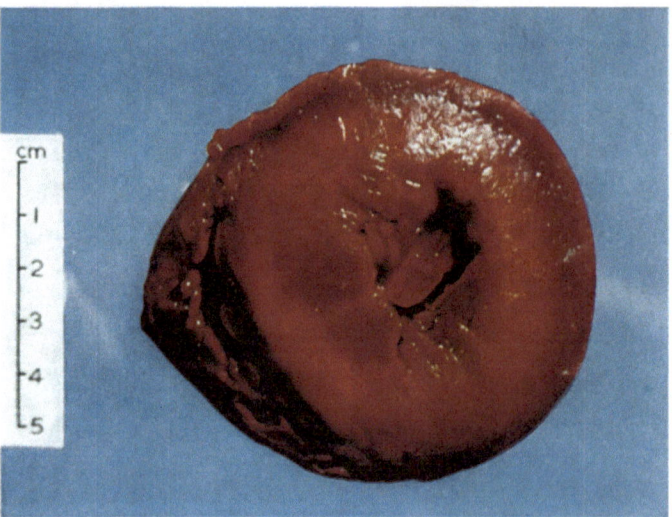

Fig. 21. A cross section through a muscle-bound left ventricle associated with aortic stenosis causing sudden death in a girl of 13 years. The right ventricle is flattened

systolic gradient exists, it should be relieved promptly without waiting for symptoms to develop. The electrocardiogram may be helpful in demonstrating the degree of ventricular hypertrophy, but the presence of a "strain" or "ischaemic" pattern (p. 57) is an indication of gross obstruction and relief should be offered if possible before this pattern appears.

Where there is regurgitation at the valves, the heart is generally better able to adapt itself to this burden at least in its initial stages. The cavity of the ventricle enlarges and the ventricular stroke volume increases. This allows for the reflux of blood which is lost with each beat, while still maintaining an adequate forward blood flow. Therefore, in the presence of regurgitation at the aortic valve, we expect to see a large heart, with a big left ventricular cavity. Some of the largest hearts occur in aortic incompetence — the so-called cor bovinum. The radiographic picture is consequently more striking than that of aortic stenosis but, as explained above, the absence of gross radiological enlargement of the heart, in the latter condition gives no grounds for complacency.

CHAPTER III

Classification of Surgical Heart Disease

A simple but complete classification of heart disease is an essential aid to differential diagnosis at the bedside. By attention to special clinical points, the diagnostic possibilities are further narrowed. Finally, special investigation may be needed to confirm or further elucidate the nature of the lesion from anatomical and physiological points of view.

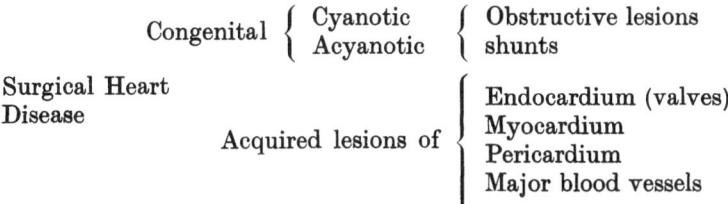

A broad distinction between congenital and acquired heart disease is generally easy to make as, for example, in uncomplicated atrial septal defect. Here the lesion has obviously been present from birth. The bulging ribs over the praecordium serve as evidence of an enlarged over-active heart from an early age, before the final moulding and adult structure of the rib cage takes place. On the other hand, conditions like isolated aortic valve stenosis continue to be a source of controversy when the lesion is discovered in middle life. There are some who believe that the calcified valve is evidence of atherosclerotic stenosis occurring in later life or as a result of rheumatic infection. Others contend that it can be explained as a congenital deformity, asymptomatic throughout early life but later, due to calcification of the deformed leaflets, it may constitute a significant and rigid obstruction. The distinction is mainly academic for the important point is to establish a diagnosis of obstruction at the aortic valve. On the other hand, mitral valve disease and aortic stenosis when they coexist, almost certainly establishes the latter condition as one of acquired rheumatic heart disease.

Cyanosis is a striking feature and generally indicates a right-to-left shunt but its presence is not always easy to determine with accuracy, particularly in infants. However, the trained observer can generally detect central cyanosis. Also the ruddy complexion common in acyanotic heart disease associated with left-to-right shunts is often striking. There is an important intermediate group in which the cyanosis is brought about by exertion. Examination for cyanosis should, therefore, always be repeated after exercise. This will unmask many unsuspected examples of communications between the pulmonary and systemic circulations.

History

While the standard schemes of history taking are likely to give all the required information, they may include a good deal of irrelevant detail and a more direct approach with some leading questions is often more productive. One's scheme of questioning will depend, to some extent, on whether the case is one of suspected congenital or acquired heart disease. Information should be deliberately sought on the following points.

1. Breathlessness
2. Haemoptysis
3. Emboli
4. Syncope
5. Angina
6. Cyanosis
7. Squatting

Breathlessness or dyspnoea is likely to be a prominent symptom. In its simplest form it represents an awareness of breathing. It may be central in origin from increased drive to the respiratory centre. More commonly in heart disease its cause lies in loss of elasticity in the lungs. These may be more turgid and more difficult to inflate because of passive congestion, as in mitral stenosis, or as a result of the actively congested and plethoric lungs of ventricular septal defect, or any other left-to-right shunt. Symptoms of dyspnoea arising from increased congestion (active or passive) are often described as "chestiness" or "recurrent bronchitis".

It is useful to fix the point at which dyspnoea appears in some simple manner; for example, the distance that can be walked on the flat or, more usefully, the number of stairs a patient can climb at a normal rate without having to rest. If a note is made of this information it is a good guide by which to judge subsequent improvement or deterioration.

Other forms of dyspnoea, such as orthopnoea and paroxysmal nocturnal dyspnoea, generally indicate a passive congestion of the lungs and are notable features of mitral stenosis and left ventricular failure. *Cough* is common in association with congested lungs and heart failure may be misinterpreted in babies with left-to-right shunts as being due to frequent "colds" or "bronchitis". On the other hand, cases of mitral stenosis with congested lungs are liable to recurrent infective bronchitis especially in the winter months.

Haemoptysis may indicate any of a number of different underlying pathological processes. Mitral stenosis is a common cause of this symptom. This may be due to bleeding from the infected congested bronchial mucosa, or from rupture of small congested capillaries. The pink blood-stained frothy sputum of pulmonary oedema is of different and more sinister significance. Patients with this symptom are in a precarious condition and relief of their obstruction is a matter of urgency.

A more alarming but probably less dangerous form of haemoptysis is the sudden coughing with little effort of a large volume of bright red blood — so-called pulmonary apoplexy. This generally occurs in cases with pulmonary venous hypertension and the sudden loss of bright red pulmonary venous blood may give temporary relief, acting as a physiological venesection.

Another cause of haemoptysis, often with pleuritic pain, is pulmonary infarction. This may result from pulmonary embolism complicating peripheral phlebothrombosis in the bed-ridden patient. Haemoptysis may also arise in cases of pulmonary arterial or venous thrombosis, where there has been a long-standing left-to-right shunt associated with pulmonary atheroma or increasing pulmonary hypertension. Pulmonary arterial thrombosis with massive infarction and haemoptysis is a classical terminal feature in cases of EISENMENGER's syndrome.

Summary of Causes of Haemoptysis

Bronchitis	Pulmonary "apoplexy"
Pulmonary congestion	Pulmonary embolism
Pulmonary oedema	Pulmonary artery thrombosis

Emboli. Embolism is common in cases with established atrial fibrillation and a past history of strokes or of vascular insufficiency in the limbs should be sought. There is a significantly increased incidence of epilepsy in patients with mitral stenosis and atrial fibrillation, and this may represent cortical scarring from earlier cerebral emboli. Rarely emboli may occur in the presence of sinus rhythm and this should arouse suspicion of bacterial endocarditis, or a friable left atrial myxoma, which may shed particles of its substance into the systemic circulation.

Syncope, or fainting, occurs classically in aortic stenosis and the cause of this on effort is not known with certainty. It may be related reflexly to the very high pressure generated in the left ventricle (in some cases over 400 mm. Hg. has been recorded).

Syncope is, however, by no means exclusively related to severe aortic stenosis. Pulmonary valve stenosis and mitral stenosis with pulmonary hypertension may give a history of syncope on exertion. These later conditions are generally associated with a fixed low cardiac output which cannot increase with exercise. A less common cause of paroxysmal fainting is the possibility of a ball-valve thrombus of the left atrium which may impact in the mitral orifice.

Angina. This occurs in many forms of surgical heart disease. If this symptom is regarded strictly as substernal pain associated with exercise, and with restricted classical paths of reference to the arm, neck, jaw and epigastrium, many cases will be overlooked. As with intermittent claudication of the calves, there is a discrepancy between the amount of blood available and the blood required by the myocardium. This may be due to a gross increase in the muscle mass, due, for example, to hypertension. In these cases angina may occur even though there is a normal coronary arterial tree. On the other hand, the coronaries may be narrowed so that they do not deliver enough blood to the muscle or, alternatively, the cardiac output may be insufficient for the heart's requirements, in spite of good muscle and coronary arteries. Several of these factors, e.g. hypertrophy, low cardiac output, and coronary disease may co-exist.

We may then expect ischaemic pain of cardiac origin with any severe stenotic lesion and the symptom can often be elicited in cases of severe mitral stenosis or of pulmonary stenosis. The pain is precipitated by exertion and relieved by rest, and may be sited over the heart itself. Whether it is actually felt there or is related to this region by the patient who is aware of "something wrong with his heart", it should be regarded as having the same significance as classical angina. Other forms of angina have been encountered and abdominal angina has been noted in children with severe aortic stenosis. The pain is felt in the epigastrium when running, and may be dismissed as a "stitch".

Cyanosis. In patients with cyanosis it is important to establish whether this has been present from birth (although it is quite frequently missed by parents in the early weeks of life), or whether it has come on at a later age. Where there is a history of cyanosis one should enquire whether the child squats, since the combination of cyanosis with squatting is characteristic of FALLOT's tetralogy.

Gross cyanosis, squatting, and cyanotic attacks, with loss of consciousness are features suggestive of pulmonary atresia (or tricuspid atresia), but where the degree of cyanosis is disproportionately great and the child is surprisingly active and not greatly incapacitated, one should suspect the possibility of transposition of the great vessels.

Cyanosis developing later in life or cyanosis coming on only with exertion is likely to be due to the late reversal of a former left-to-right shunt as, in the EISENMENGER group of conditions. Again, one should keep in mind the condition of ventricular septal defect with moderate pulmonary stenosis (so-called "acyanotic" FALLOT).

Family and Past History

In congenital heart disease a family history of heart disease may be relevant. Congenital heart disease of the same type may occur in identical twins. Enquiry may reveal a past history of rheumatic fever, chorea, scarlet fever or severe tonsillitis, though this is by no means invariable in cases of rheumatic heart disease. A history of maternal rubella in early pregnancy can be of considerable importance in congenital heart disease in an infant.

Physical Examination

General. The paramount importance of a thorough examination at the bedside cannot be over-emphasized. In general, a careful, intelligent physical examination will yield a good deal more information than long detailed histories and elaborate investigations.

The patient should be at ease on a firm couch or high hospital bed and with the head and shoulders raised at an angle of about 30 degrees. If the patient is on a low bed, the doctor should sit on a chair at the patient's side. The room should be warm if one is to assess degrees of cyanosis, the state of the peripheral circulation and the pulses. The legs and toes must be accessible for inspection and palpation.

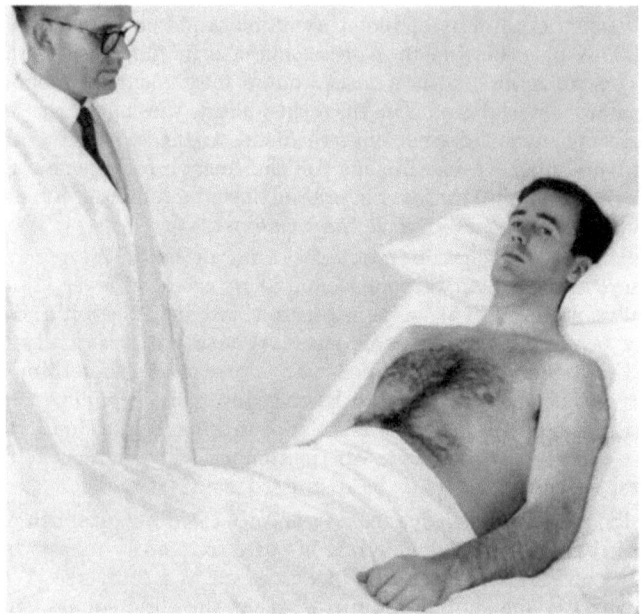

Fig. 22. Patient in position for examination at an angle of about 30°, relaxed and in a good light

Little of definite value can be learned from the general physical build, but bulging and deformity of the chest in the region of the praecordium may provide a clue to the presence of a congenital heart lesion and, quite frequently, patients with ventricular septal defect have a prominent sternum. Patients with severe mitral disease are often thin and have a cyanotic malar flush; with associated tricuspid disease there may be, in addition, brown pigmentation of the skin.

Characteristically, cases of atrial septal defect are said to have a small-boned gracile build, with long tapering fingers and a high-arched palate, but this is certainly not an invariable picture. On the other hand, patients with pulmonary valve stenosis and a closed ventricular septum may have a rounded "moon face" and highly-coloured cheeks.

Cyanosis. A patient may be obviously cyanosed, doubtfully cyanosed, of normal colour, or may have a complexion suggestive of a left-to-right shunt. Central cyanosis suggests the presence of a right-to-left intracardiac shunt, while red cheeks and bright red lips may indicate a left-to-right shunt. Cyanosis is caused by the presence of reduced haemoglobin visible in the vessels of the skin and mucous membranes and may be peripheral or central in distribution. We are not much concerned with the former, which is present in a number of conditions with inadequate peripheral circulation. Central cyanosis is best detected in the "warm" areas, lips, conjunctivae, and tongue.

In general, the presence of central cyanosis indicates the mixing of venous and arterial blood within the heart or major arteries, but one should keep in mind the possibility of cyanosis due to other conditions, such as lung disease, pulmonary arterio-venous fistula, sulphaemoglobinuria and the blue dyes.

It is convenient to record the degree of cyanosis noted according to a simple grading. This enables one to judge deterioration or improvement, particularly in the FALLOT group of conditions. Four grades of severity can be distinguished.

Grade I. This is cyanosis on exertion only; e.g. the patient having a ventricular septal defect and a mild degree of pulmonary stenosis which does not cause shunting unless combined with the fall of systemic resistance accompanying exercise. On the other hand it may indicate commencing reversal of a predominantly left-to-right shunt due to increasing pulmonary vascular resistence. Under this sub-heading of Grade I cyanosis on exertion, one must be on the look out for the interesting and significant feature of *differential cyanosis*. This can mean cyanosis of the lower extremities with a normal pink colour of the arms and face. It may be present at rest but is more likely to be brought on by exertion. It generally indicates a reversal of blood flow through a persistent ductus arteriosus as a result of pulmonary hypertension. Poorly oxygenated pulmonary arterial blood then mixes with that of the descending aorta supplying the lower limbs. As the pulmonary resistance rises progressively, more pulmonary arterial blood is shunted into the aorta and eventually flows proximally into the aortic arch, giving a variety of bizarre colour combinations.

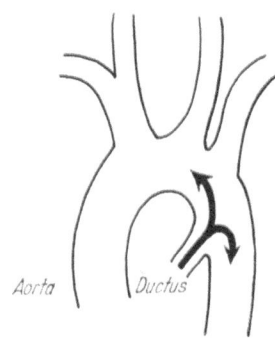

Fig. 23. With the reversal of blood flow through a ductus, desaturated blood is directed to the lower half of the body and possibly to the left arm

For example, one could have cyanosis of the feet and left hand together with the left half of the face as well.

Grade II. This is cyanosis of a mild degree which is, as a rule, only detectable to a trained observer. The patient is often not regarded as being abnormally coloured by the casual observer.

Grade III. This degree of cyanosis is obvious to the lay observer and includes most cases of recognisable cyanotic heart disease.

Grade IV. This is cyanosis or blueness of a gross degree, commonly seen in severely disabled cases of FALLOT's tetralogy, pulmonary and tricuspid atresia, transposition of the great vessels and the terminal phases of reversed shunts.

Clubbing. An examination of the fingers for clubbing should be part of the routine inspection of the hands preliminary to feeling the pulses. One generally also feels the patient's hands to gain some estimate of the peripheral systemic blood flow; in conditions of low-cardiac output they will be cold and the patient complains of cold hands and feet. Attention should next be directed to the toes to assess the degree of clubbing and the peripheral circulation there. As with differential cyanosis there may be differential clubbing of the toes in cases of persistent ductus arteriosus with reversed shunt.

The mechanism of production of clubbing remains obscure. It is common in a large number of conditions, particularly suppurative lung disease, and bronchial carcinoma. It may occur as part of the condition of pulmonary hypertrophic osteoarthropathy. Clubbing may be mediated through the presence in the blood of a vaso-dilating factor, either arising as a secretion in the lungs or from failure of the lungs to "remove" such a substance produced elsewhere. This could explain its presence in lung diseases and also in conditions of right-to-left shunts where a portion of the blood flow by-passes the lungs.

It is convenient to grade the degree of clubbing noted.

Grade I. There is a filling in of the angle between the nail and the nail-bed. The latter is shiny and prominent.

Grade II. In addition to the above features there is a "watch-glass" contour of the nails with convexity in two planes, longitudinal as well as lateral.

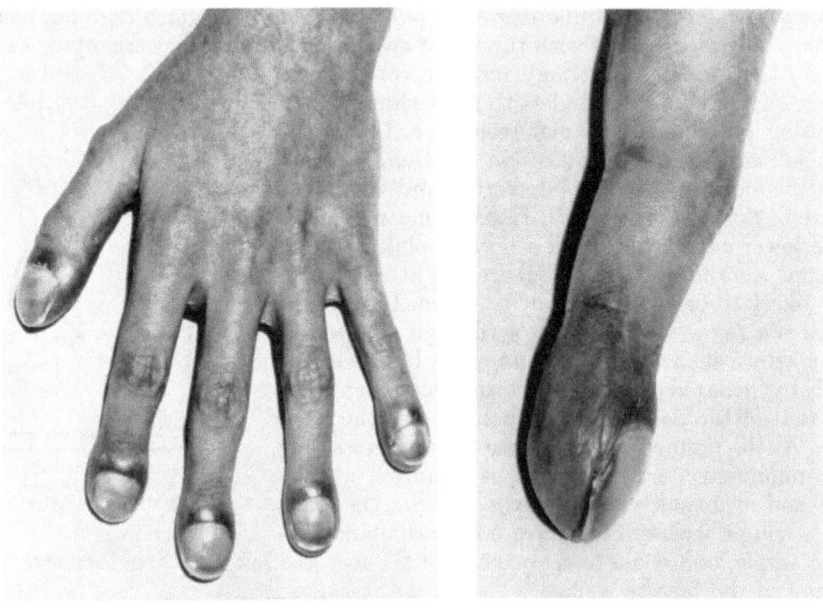

Fig. 24. Severe grade V clubbing demonstrating all the above features

Grade III. There is an increase in the volume of the soft tissue digital pulp in addition to the above features.

Grade IV. This is an exaggerated stage of the above, with swelling of the tissues on each side of the nail-bed.

Grade V. This is revealed as gross "drum-stick" formation of the ends of the digits, and may be associated with clubbing of the nose.

Oedema. During the general inspection and assessment of the patient before examining the cardiovascular system more specifically, it is convenient to feel for pitting oedema of the ankles as a sign of raised systemic venous pressure or right heart decompensation. Firm, maintained pressure for 15—30 seconds is necessary to detect minor pitting, and pressure should be against a firm background as, for example, the subcutaneous border of the tibia.

Keep in mind the fact that ankle oedema is unlikely in patients confined to bed. In these cases it is the sacral area which must be inspected, and digital pressure here will often reveal a considerable sacral pad of oedema. Where there is evidence of much fluid retention, evidence of ascites and an enlarged liver should be sought.

CHAPTER IV

Examination of the Cardiovascular System

In examining the heart itself one is trying to evaluate the efficiency of two pumps working side by side. Consequently, we look into the question of the output of the pumps (arterial pulses), their ability to cope with their input of blood (venous pressure and pulse) and feel for evidence of over-activity of one or other "pump". In addition we may detect turbulence as the blood passes through narrow or irregular channels (thrills).

Having made an assessment of the nature of the disorder and its most likely site, it is then useful to listen to the working of the pump in different areas, in order to gain more accurate information.

The Pulses

The arterial pulse gives information about the rate and regularity of the heart's action and, more important, gives some indication of the output of the left ventricle. One can derive additional information from the form of the pulse wave. For example, in aortic stenosis the pulse may have a slow rise and a sustained "plateau" character.

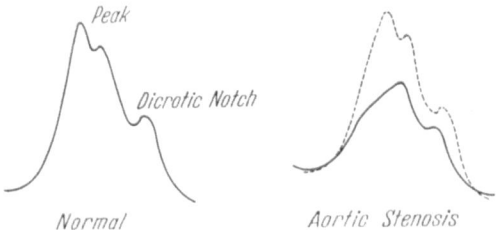

Fig. 25. Figures show the normal pulse contour and the alterations brought about by aortic stenosis

In examining the pulses it is important to examine as many as possible, certainly both radial and both femoral pulses. In this way a diagnosis of coarctation of the aorta can be made immediately. In a man with absent femoral pulses one should next feel for the aortic pulse in the epigastrium. If this is present and the femorals are absent, the diagnosis is likely to be aortic thrombosis (LERICHE syndrome) and not coarctation.

It is a help in feeling the femoral pulse to have the feet in maximal external rotation. This brings the femoral artery forward over the head of the femur.

Examination of the peripheral pulses is important in cases of mitral stenosis with atrial fibrillation, as it may provide the only evidence of systemic embolism.

The examination of the arm pulse should not be confined to the radial, which is often small and difficult to evaluate, whereas the brachial pulse may be more helpful. Palpation of the carotid pulse in the neck should not be omitted. This pulse is often visible and palpation will help to distinguish it from venous pulsation. In addition, it is frequently possible to feel a thrill transmitted to the neck vessels from the aortic arch while feeling the carotid artery.

A bounding pulse easily visible in the neck and clearly perceptible on palpation should raise the possibilities of persistent ductus arteriosus, coarctation, or aortic incompetence.

Disturbances of rhythm (atrial fibrillation, paroxysmal tachycardia, etc.) do not, as a rule, fall within the scope of a surgical textbook, but a number of cha-

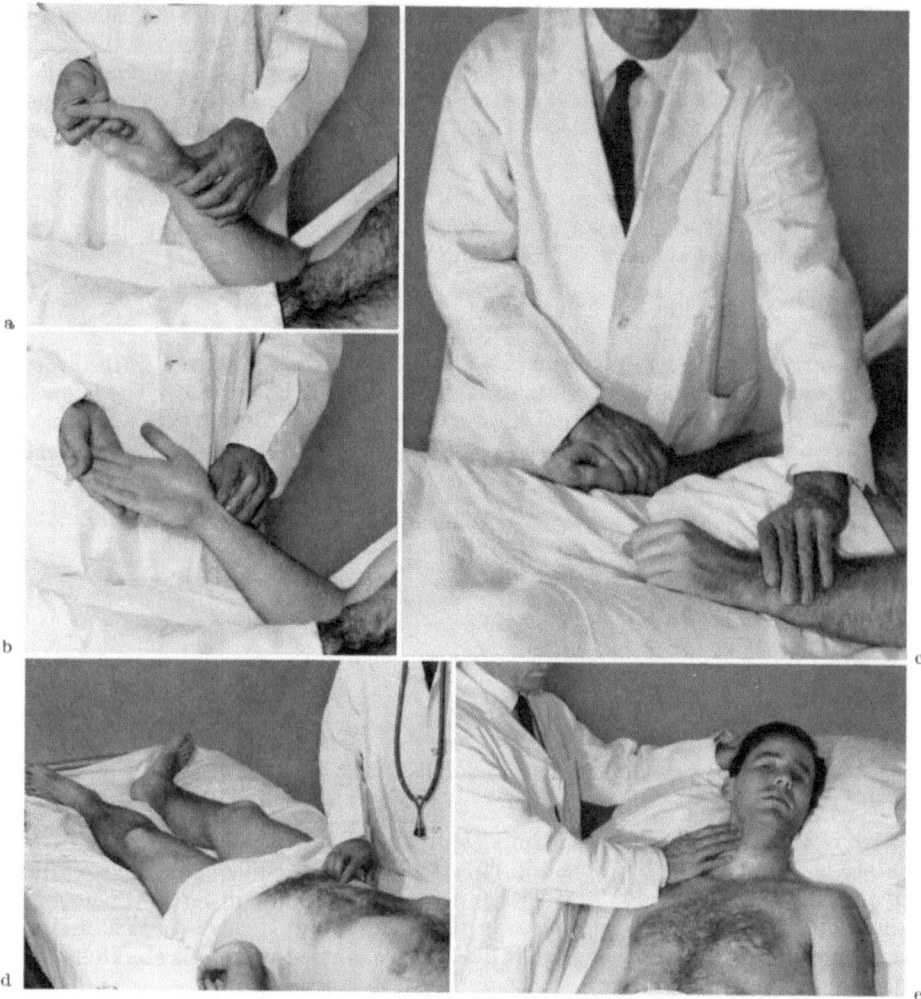

Fig. 26a—e. a The arterial pulse. While feeling the radial pulse the fingers are inspected. They give an indication of the peripheral circulation and the nails are examined for clubbing. b While examining the pulse, the palm is inspected for the diffuse redness associated with hepatic dysfunction. c Both radial pulses should be felt and compared synchronously. d In feeling for the femoral pulses the feet should be in external rotation. e The carotid pulse may give valuable information with regard to the pulse contour and associated thrills in the carotid artery will be felt

racteristic pulse irregularities have been described and are commonly encountered in surgical practice.

Pulsus bigeminus. This is a disturbance of rhythm where the impulses are coupled. The coupled beats represent a normal pulse followed by an extrasystole and each pair is followed by a compensatory pause. Pulsus bigeminus may be a sign of digitalis intoxication (p. 53).

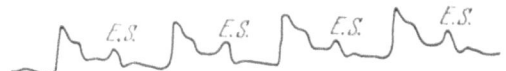

Fig. 27. Pulse tracing showing pulsus bigeminus. Each normal beat is followed by an extrasystole and a compensatory pause

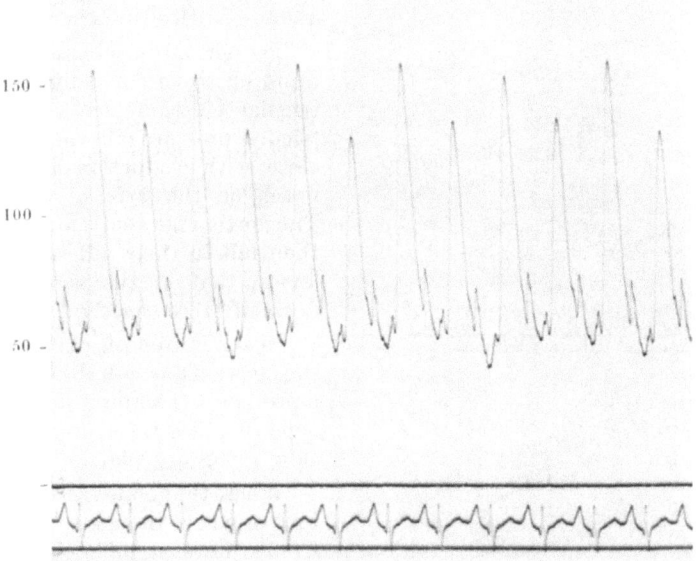

Fig. 28. Pulse contour in a case of pulsus alternans. Each succeeding beat has a reduced force

Pulsus alternans is a disturbance of force. Here each alternate beat is of reduced force or amplitude. It may be of serious prognostic significance and generally indicates left ventricular failure, resulting, for example, from hypertension or aortic stenosis.

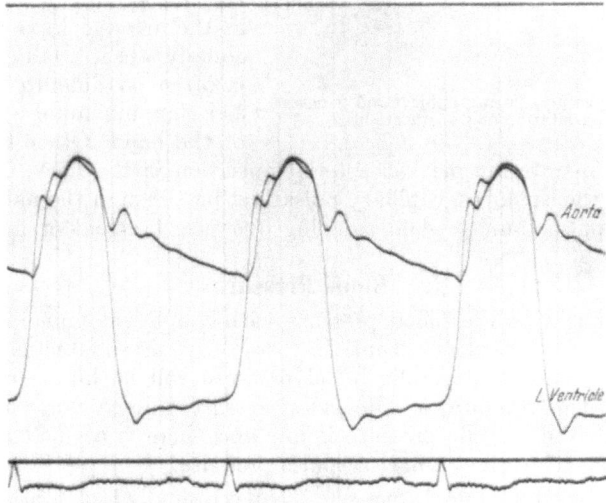

Fig. 29. This shows synchronous pressure tracings from the left ventricle and aorta

Pulsus paradoxus. In normal circumstances, a deep inspiration, by reducing intrathoracic pressure, increases the venous return to the heart. This increased filling of the right ventricle results in an increased output (STARLING's law), but in constrictive pericarditis diastolic filling of the heart is limited by the pericardium so that the output of the heart (and hence the pulse volume) does not increase with inspiration.

The **normal pulse** has a moderately rapid upstroke coinciding with ventricular ejection. As the left ventricular pressure falls the aortic valve closes with production of the dicrotic notch on the arterial downstroke. The aortic and ventricular pressures then fall to their different diastolic levels, that in the ventricle being normally zero (fig. 29).

In aortic stenosis of severe degree the ejection phase of the left ventricle is prolonged. This produces a flattened type of pulse wave — the so-called slow rising or "plateau" pulse.

Where the aortic valve is incompetent or where there is a leak of blood from the systemic circulation in diastole, for example through a persistent ductus arteriosus, there will be an abrupt fall of pressure in diastole to an abnormally low level. This is the so-called collapsing or CORRIGAN pulse. There results also an increased left ventricular stroke volume, producing a rapid upstroke in the arterial wave form with an equally abrupt fall of pressure. It is often possible to feel this pulse as a slapping impulse against the flat of the hand. Other features of this

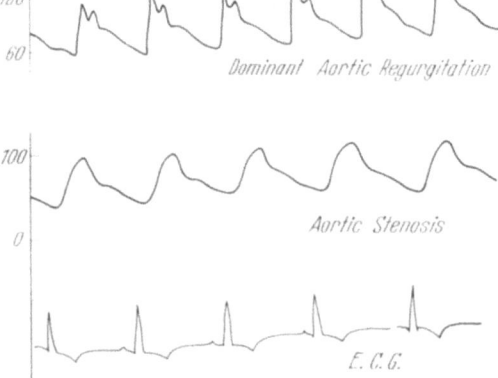

Fig. 30. Pulse curves in a normal subject and in cases of aortic regurgitation and aortic stenosis

haemodynamic state are marked arterial pulsation in the neck, sometimes with movement of the ear lobes, capillary pulsation, best seen in the nail beds and lips and audible pulse sounds when listening over the brachial or femoral arteries.

Blood Pressure

The assessment of the blood pressure with a sphygmomanometer is part of the evaluation of the cardiac output. In cases of persistent ductus arteriosus and aortic incompetence the systolic blood pressure will be high and the diastolic pressure low. This produces a wide *pulse pressure*. The converse occurs in aortic stenosis where the systolic pressure is low and there is a small fall in pressure during diastole. This gives a narrow pulse pressure.

Where the blood pressure in the arms is unexpectedly high, one should consider the possibility of coarctation of the aorta and feel the femoral pulses. On the other hand, where one has made a diagnosis of coarctation and the systemic blood pressure is lower than one would have anticipated, it is well to remember the possibility of coarctation with associated aortic stenosis.

The assessment of blood pressure at half-hourly intervals is of great value in the post-operative management of a cardiac surgical case, in helping to assess shock and haemorrhage. It can also be of value in the early detection of systemic embolism within the arterial tree. For example, after mitral valvotomy a rise in blood pressure may be suggestive of embolism and in an unconscious patient may be the first sign before evidence of ischaemia or loss of function, in the area of occlusion.

After closure of a persistent ductus arteriosus, there is a narrowing of the pulse pressure as the result of the closure of the fistulous leak. In coarctation the blood pressure does not fall immediately postoperatively, emphasising that the mechanical obstruction of the aorta is not the only factor maintaining the high blood pressure. The pressure generally falls slowly over a period of one to three weeks.

The Venous Pulse

This may give a great deal of information and is best studied in the neck. The patient should be sitting up at an angle of about 30 degrees, and with a good and movable light source for tangential lighting.

The first observation to be made is the level of the venous *pressure* by noting the height to which the veins are distended above the level of the right atrium.

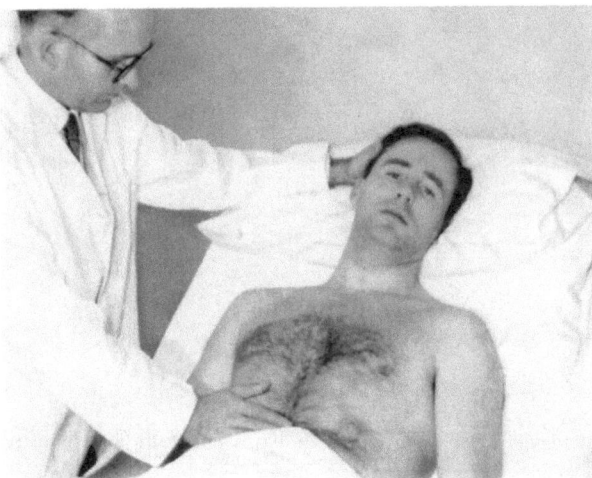

Fig. 31. For inspection of the jugular pulse the neck muscles should be relaxed. Pressure exerted with the right hand over the liver will elicit the hepato-jugular reflux

Then the right hand should compress the region of the liver or right hypochondrium. This increases the venous pressure and distends the external jugular vein — the so-called hepato-jugular reflux. This manoeuvre also helps to emphasize venous pulsation and, at the same time, gives an indication of the size and tenderness of the liver.

The next feature to study is the venous *pulsation*, and to distinguish it from arterial pulsation. Apart from the position of the pulse in the line of the veins — venous pulsation has a rapid flicking quality unlike arterial pulsation. Also venous waves are more easily seen than felt — arterial waves vice versa.

Normally, three waves are detected, *a*, *c*, and *v*, and they can be most conveniently timed by listening to the heart sounds with a stethoscope while observing these waves. The *a* wave just precedes the first heart sound and the *v* follows the second sound.

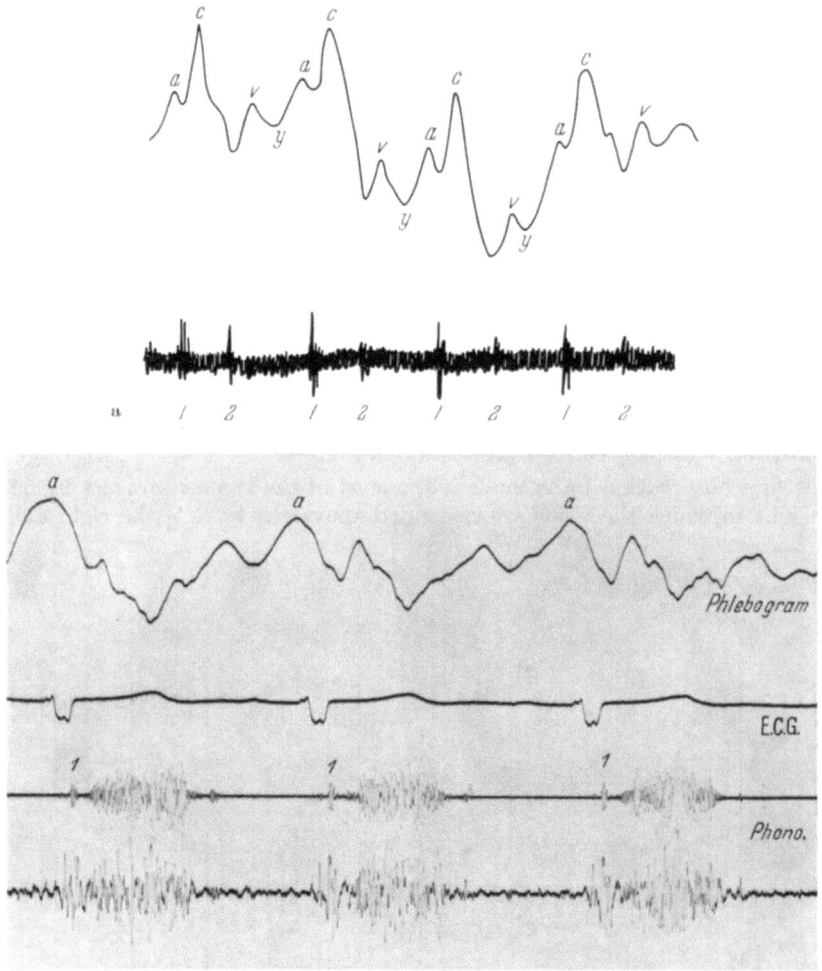

Fig. 32 a and b. The jugular phlebogram (a) shown diagrammatically and (b) in relation to the heart sounds in a case of pulmonary stenosis

In addition to the above *a*, *c*, and *v* waves, two negative waves or pressure deflections are described — *x* and *y*.

The a wave is due to atrial contraction which briefly increases intra-atrial pressure. It is, therefore, absent in atrial fibrillation.

The c wave. There has been a good deal of controversy regarding the *c* wave, so-called because it is co-incident with the carotid pulse and, therefore, synchronous with ventricular systole. It is not, only, due to the carotid pulse in the neck, as can be demonstrated by its presence in cardiac catheterization pressures recorded from the right atrium. One explanation is that it arises from a billowing of the tricuspid valve cusps into the atrium. This is brought about by the rise of ventricular pressure during systole.

The x descent. During ventricular contraction the atrioventricular ring is pulled down by the concentric contraction of the ventricles. This reduces the right atrial pressure and in this way produces the negative deflection following the *c* wave.

The v wave. With the tricuspid valve firmly closed throughout the systole, blood continues to flow from both venae cavae into the right atrium which is then

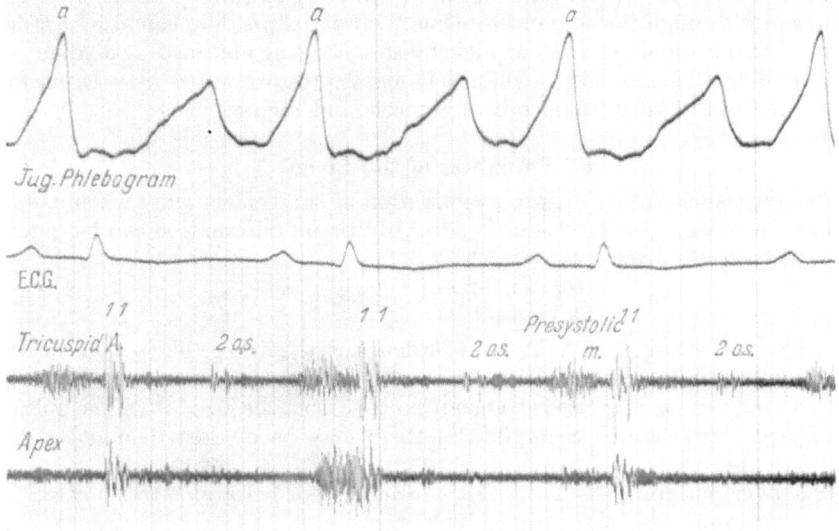

Fig. 33. Giant "a" waves in a case of tricuspid stenosis

virtually a closed chamber. There is, consequently, a progressive rise of right atrial pressure producing a positive *v* wave.

The y descent. The ventricle relaxes, the pulmonary valve closes and the right ventricular pressure falls. When this falls below the right atrial pressure the tricuspid valve opens and there is a rapid fall of right atrial pressure as blood pours from atrium to ventricle. This fall of pressure produces the *y* descent.

In the presence of *tricuspid stenosis*, the right atrial pressure will be high and there will be a high pressure throughout the venous system. Also, with normal rhythm, there will be an increased force of right atrial contraction producing large *a* waves. In addition, the rate of the *y* descent will be slow since the blood can escape only slowly across the narrow valve orifice into the right ventricle during diastole.

Giant a waves, representing a high pressure in the right atrium can occur from any cause of obstruction to right atrial emptying. Thus tricuspid stenosis or diminished distensibility of the right ventricle due to right ventricular hypertrophy, pulmonary hypertension or pulmonary stenosis may be the cause of this. Right ventricular filling resistance may also be increased by septal hypertrophy either as an isolated condition or as part of *left* ventricular (and septal) hypertrophy — BERNHEIM phenomenon.

Giant v waves: In tricuspid regurgitation there will be a reflux of blood into the right atrium during systole with a rise of pressure in that chamber co-incident with systole. These reflux systolic waves are giant *v* waves. Large *v* waves have been described in atrial septal defect, particularly in children, due to exaggerated filling of the right atrium against a closed tricuspid valve. This filling is not only from the vena cava but also from the left atrium.

Cannon waves occur characteristically in complete heart block. In these circumstances there is dissociation between atrial and ventricular contractions. When atrial and ventricular contractions coincide, the right atrium contracts against a closed tricuspid valve producing a steep rise of pressure in the jugular veins.

A venous wave pattern identical with that found in the right atrium can be recorded from the left atrium either by direct puncture of that chamber at operation or through the skin or bronchus. Left atrial pressure can also be studied indirectly from the pulmonary capillary venous tracing obtained at cardiac catheterization (p. 61). A study of these left atrial pressure waves may be useful in diagnosing and distinguishing mitral stenosis and regurgitation.

Palpation of the Liver

The liver is felt as part of the examination of the venous pulse when one tries to elicit the hepato-jugular reflux (p. 29). Additional information can be obtained with regard to the liver   (a) size
                                                  (b) tenderness
                                                  (c) pulsation

In right heart failure or right heart obstruction the liver is likely to be enlarged and may be painful and tender as a result of distension of its capsule. Where a fluctuating venous pressure is transmitted to it from the heart it will be pulsatile. In tricuspid stenosis and regurgitation there may be marked liver pulsation in time with the venous pulse.

True liver pulsation should be distinguished from pulsations transmitted from the ventricles or aorta through the liver.

Inspection of the Praecordium

Note should be made of the form and the movement of the praecordium.

(a) **Form.** Bulging of the chest wall in the region of the heart may point to a congenital lesion suggesting that the heart was enlarged and perhaps over-active from an early age — before firm moulding and ossification of the ribs took place. Cases of pure ventricular septal defect with raised pulmonary flow and resistance commonly have a prominent narrow sternum (pigeon chest).

(b) **Movements.** Areas of pulsation often indicate an active left ventricle if confined to the apex, or over-activity of the right ventricle and its outflow tract may be noted along the left sternal border. Again, an active hyperdynamic praecordial impulse is suggestive of an intracardiac shunt with large volumes of blood pouring through the right ventricular outflow and pulmonary artery. On the other hand, obstructive lesions of the heart are more often associated with a slower, more sustained type of pulsation. These features are more apparent on palpation of the heart.

Palpation of the Ventricles

This is one of the most important aspects of the clinical examination of the heart. By this means it should be possible to assess which ventricle carries the burden of the cardiac lesion and, also, the nature of this burden.

One, therefore, examines for evidence of:

(a) which ventricle is under strain, and

(b) whether the load is obstructive in nature or is due to an increased stroke volume.

The **left ventricular impulse** is normally felt at the apex of the heart in the region of the left nipple or just below the left breast in a woman.

The area of impulse against the ribs and intercostal space is generally localised and is often visible on inspection. In standard schemes of cardiological examination the "apex beat" is usually carefully noted in relation to the ribs and its distance from the mid-line. But this position can vary widely, depending upon underlying lung disease, fluid, position of the diaphragm, physical build, etc. Any of these features may result in displacement of the apex beat apart from that resulting from cardiac enlargement. The assessment of the *nature* of the left ventricular impulse is of far greater value than a description of its position.

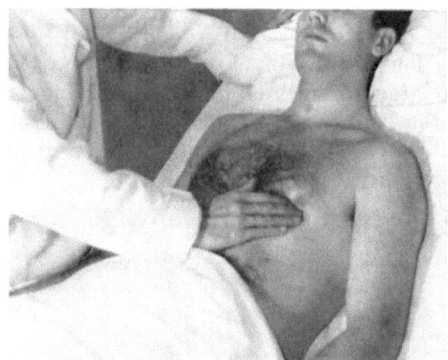

Fig. 34. The position of the left ventricular impulse is located

Where the left ventricle is *obstructed*, as in aortic stenosis, it will be hypertrophied and will transmit a localised but powerful heaving and sustained type of impulse to the flat of the hand. Where the left ventricle is pumping *extra volumes* of blood, as in ventricular septal defect, persistent ductus arteriosus, or aortic incompetence, the impulse from the now enlarged left ventricle may be diffuse, but its character will be more active, turbulent, and hyperdynamic (as opposed to the sustained heave of obstruction).

Similar observations apply to the *right ventricle*. The **right ventricular impulse** is palpable to the left of the sternum in the third and fourth interspaces, and again, is felt best with the flat of the hand.

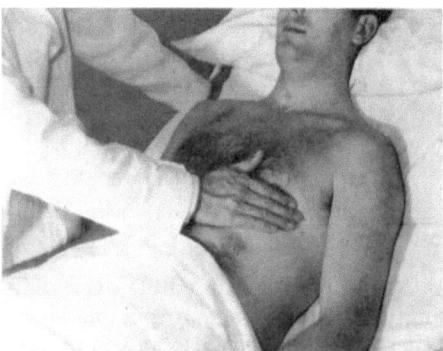

Fig. 35. Evaluation of left ventricular activity — force and character of the impulse

As with left ventricular lesions, obstructive lesions of the right ventricle result in a sustained heave but over a rather wider area than that of the left ventricular impulse. This is best illustrated in pulmonary valve stenosis with closed ventricular septum, but can be appreciated in many cases of increased pressure in the right ventricle. Where the right ventricle ejects an increased volume of blood it is dilated and over-active so that one will again feel a diffuse and turbulent impulse over the region of the right ventricular outflow.

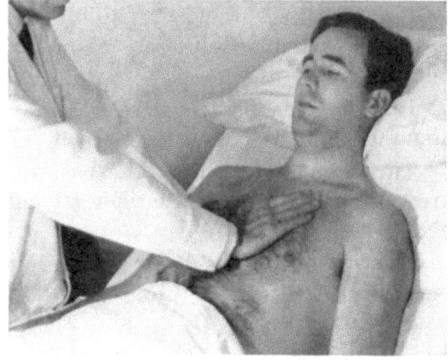

Fig. 36. The right ventricular impulse is felt along the left sternal border

This is best illustrated in atrial septal defect. In these cases the dilated and pulsating pulmonary artery may sometimes be felt in addition over the second left interspace.

In assessing the work of the right or left ventricle it is again convenient to grade it according to the degree of over-activity (load or volume work). This can be done on an arbitrary scale of 0 to + + + + If the assessment is made by the same observer on each examination, this information can be used to judge clinical improvement or deterioration.

Thrills and Palpable "Sounds"

The passage of blood through narrow segments or, alternatively, the passage of large volumes of blood through normal channels, is liable to give rise to an intensively turbulent blood flow. This turbulence can be appreciated as a palpable vibration, or if less intense, may be manifest only as a murmur.

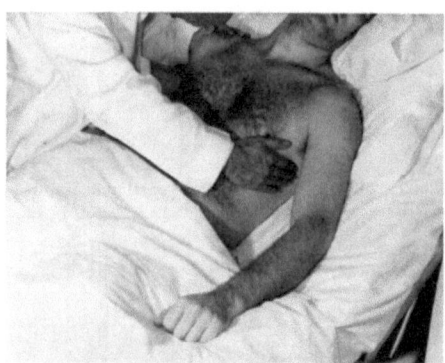 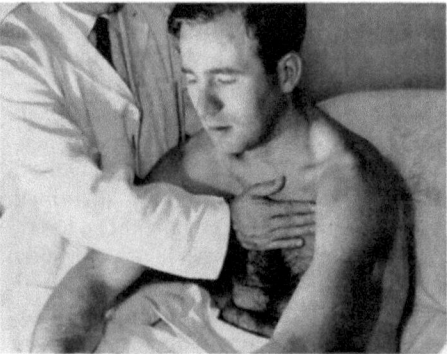

Fig. 37   Fig. 38

Fig. 37. In feeling for mitral thrills the patient should be rolled slightly over towards the left

Fig. 38. Thrills emanating from the aortic and pulmonary valves are best felt with the patient sitting up and with the breath held in expiration

Murmurs may be audible over wide areas of the praecordium and the site of maximum loudness may not be easy to determine. The palpable thrill, on the other hand is less diffuse and is of great value in localising the probable site of the lesion giving rise to the turbulence.

In this way, obstructions at the aortic, mitral or pulmonary valves are often localised with accuracy, by palpating a thrill in the appropriate area; while the murmur (particularly in aortic stenosis) is likely to be widely conducted throughout the praecordium.

In feeling for thrills, one should bear in mind that the diastolic thrill of mitral stenosis is felt best with the patient rolled slightly over to the left.

Thrills emanating from the base of the heart (aortic and pulmonary valves) are best felt with the patient sitting forward and with the breath held in expiration.

The thrills of infundibular stenosis and of ventricular septal defect are generally best felt in the third and fourth left interspaces respectively.

Closure of the cardiac valves gives rise to the heart sounds but the shock waves they produce are not generally palpable.

On the other hand, where the valve closure is forceful and under increased pressure, the vibrations of the "closing sound" can often be detected by the examining hand. Thus, in mitral stenosis the loud first sound or "closing snap" of the mitral valve may be felt in these patients at the apex; and in conditions of severe pulmonary hypertension, the forceful closure of the pulmonary valve can sometimes be felt over the base of the heart.

Summary Illustrating Some of the Foregoing Points in Clinical Diagnosis

One may encounter a young woman patient with a history of breathlessness on exertion. Her pulses are small in volume and possibly reveal atrial fibrillation. The extremities are cold, suggesting a reduced cardiac output. There may be increased jugular venous pulsation with a dominant a wave.

Inspection of the praecordium reveals a slight heave to the left of the sternum. On palpation this is of a sustained nature in the distribution of the right ventricle and with the severity of $+$ to $++$. At the same time, one can appreciate a palpable second "sound" over the base of the heart, suggesting, with the right ventricular heave, that the pulmonary artery pressure is raised. On palpation at the apex no left ventricular thrust or overactivity can be felt but the slapping first "sound" may be palpable and a thrill can be felt as the cardiac impulse recedes from the hand in diastole.

These findings can be summarised thus: small regular pulse, cold periphery.

a wave
R. V. $++$ L. V. O.
M_1 and P_2 palpable. Diastolic thrill at apex.

We now know without recourse to the stethoscope that this young lady probably has mitral stenosis with some increase of her pulmonary artery pressure (pulmonary hypertension) as revealed by the over-active right ventricle, a wave, and palpable pulmonary valve closure. The stethoscope can now be used as it should be used — in order to confirm one's previous findings, and to assess them with more accuracy. In this case it is *not* being used to make the diagnosis.

In other words, one should know what to listen *for* on the basis of information available from inspection and palpation. Listening first is not the surest way to a diagnosis, since the sensitive ear will give us too much auditory information. On the other hand, with the clinical information already available we can listen selectively and in that way derive a maximum of useful information from the clinical use of the senses.

In the example above we know we shall hear a loud mitral first sound (which was palpable) and we know we shall hear a rumbling diastolic murmur as revealed by the thrill. We shall quickly note these features and listen more selectively and carefully for an opening snap of the mitral valve, suggesting its pliability, and for the blowing systolic murmur which may suggest associated mitral or tricuspid regurgitation. Likewise, at the base we expect a loud pulmonary second sound due to pulmonary hypertension and we listen carefully for possible basal diastolic murmurs of, say, pulmonary regurgitation — the turbulence of which is not generally palpable.

Auscultation of the Heart

As has been suggested above, the stethoscope can be most usefully employed in listening for specific features and should not be regarded as the primary tool for making a diagnosis.

Accurate auscultation can elicit a great deal of information once the mechanism underlying the sounds and murmurs is understood. Consequently, the emphasis in the following section is on an explanation of the "mechanics" of the auditory phenomena. Thereafter, facility and skill in the use of the stethoscope will follow with diligence and an intelligent application of the ear. The attitude of "listening hopefully" for a diagnosis to present itself should be avoided.

Heart sounds. Two clearly defined sounds can be distinguished in each cardiac cycle and are readily heard over the whole praecordium. The gap between the first and second sound represents the systolic phase of the cardiac cycle, and the rather longer gap before the next first sound represents diastole. Third and fourth heart sounds can be heard in certain circumstances by the trained observer. A number of additional sounds can sometimes be heard.

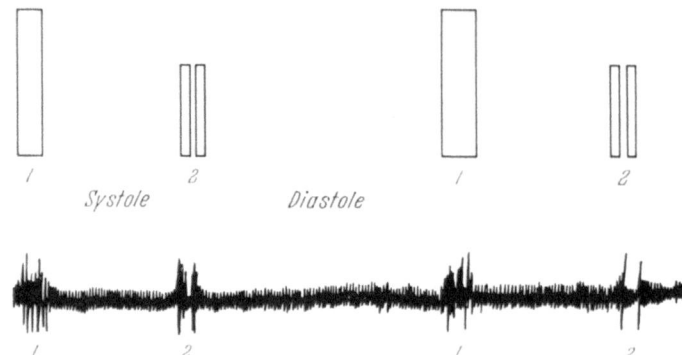

Fig. 39. Diagrammatic representation of the first and second heart sounds

The First Heart Sound. This is probably caused almost wholly by the closure of the mitral and tricuspid valves. Since it is the rule for the electrical and mechanical events of the left side of the heart to precede fractionally those of the right, the valves close asynchronously. Under normal conditions, mitral valve closure thus precedes tricuspid valve closure. The first sound is, therefore, normally split into two components, the first component being due to closure of the mitral valve and the second is due to closure of the tricuspid valve. This split of the first sound is not always clearly heard with the stethoscope, but it is a normal phenomenon and can be distinguished on the phonocardiogram. The first sound is heard most clearly when listening over the mitral and tricuspid areas of the heart. Its rather lower pitch compared with the second sound is said to be due to the muscular component of the sound.

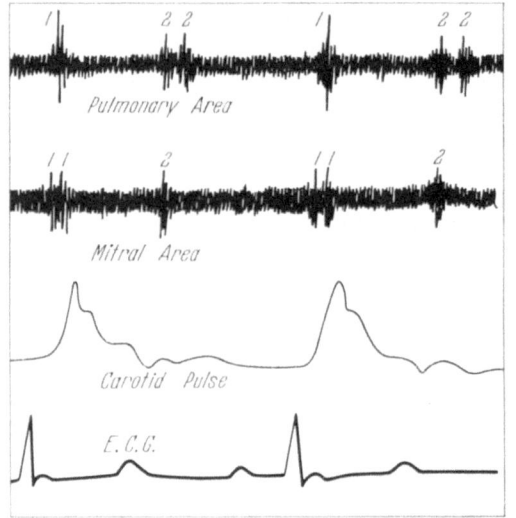

Fig. 40. Idealised figure representing the split of the first sound at the mitral area and the split second sound at the pulmonary area

The Second Heart Sound. This is most clearly heard over the base of the heart and is due to the closure of the aortic and pulmonary valves. As with the first sound, left heart events precede those of the right so that the second sound also is normally split, the aortic component (A_2) preceding that of the pulmonary (P_2). This splitting of the second sound at the base is easily heard in most normal people and is particularly conspicuous in children.

A characteristic feature of the second sound is the variation in the splitting of the components with respiration. Normally, with inspiration there is increased filling of the right heart with blood, so that the ejection phase of the right ventricle is prolonged. As a result pulmonary valve closure is further delayed, and splitting of the sound is therefore widened. On expiration the splitting again narrows.

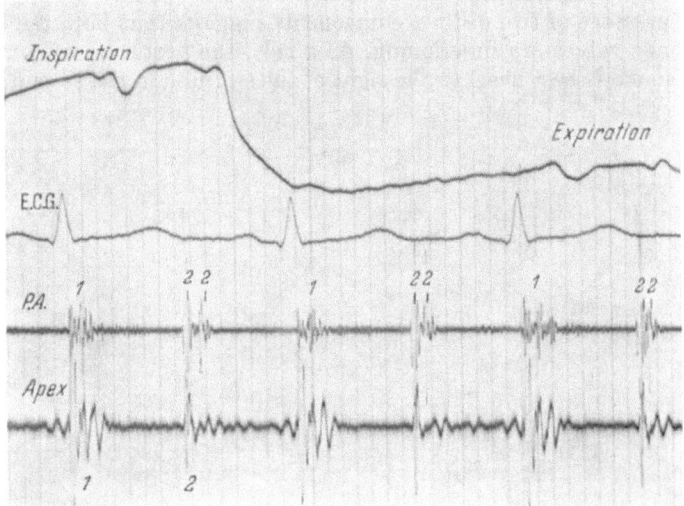

Fig. 41. Phonocardiographic tracing showing: a) The composite nature of the first sound at the apex. b) The splitting of the second sound at the pulmonary area. c) The respiratory variation of the second sound

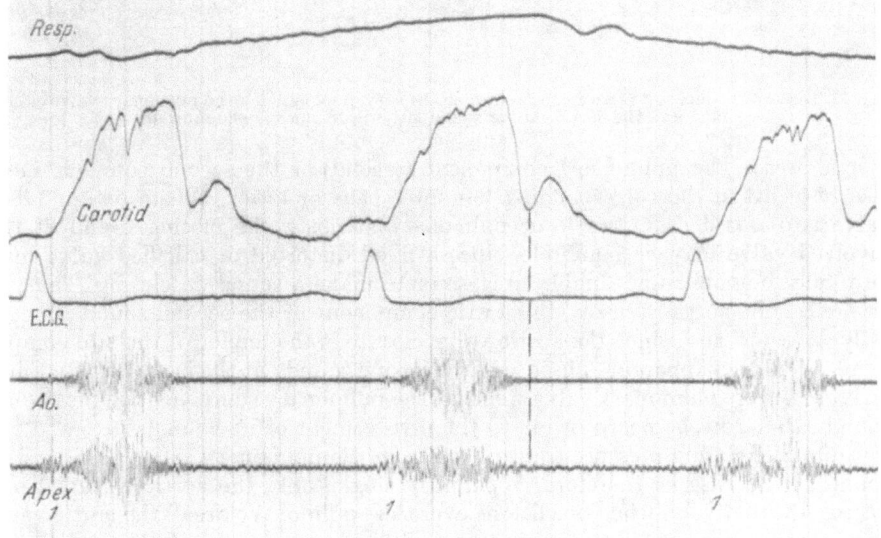

Fig. 42. Phonocardiogram from a case of aortic stenosis showing an "absence" of the second sound which should correspond with the notch of the carotid trace

In general, the two components of the second heart sound are best heard with the patient sitting up. In order to elicit this variation of splitting with respiration, the patient should then be instructed to breathe rhythmically and quietly through the open mouth.

In listening critically to the second heart sound the following information should be noted.

(a) The presence of two distinct components

(b) The width and variation of the interval between components with respiration, and

(c) the loudness of the separate components of the sound.

(a) The **presence of two distinct components** suggests that both the aortic and the pulmonary valves are functioning. As a rule, the aortic (first) component of the second sound is best heart to the right of the sternum in the second interspace

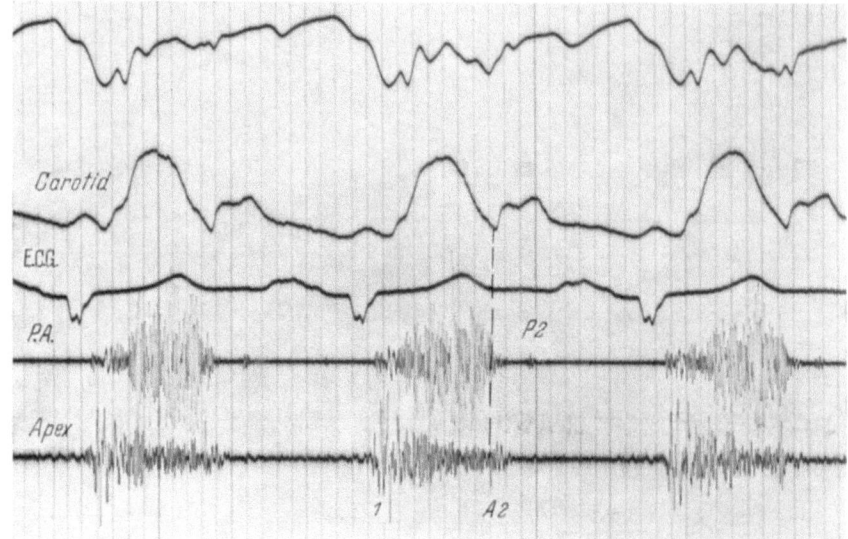

Fig. 43. A case of pulmonary valve stenosis showing the very quiet and delayed pulmonary valve closing sound and the aortic closing sound lost within the systolic murmur

(aortic area). The pulmonary component (second) of the second sound is most clearly heard in the corresponding left interspace or lower. Where one or other valve is diseased as in aortic or pulmonary stenosis, the closing sound of the involved valve may be inaudible, since a fixed distorted or calcified valve may be totally immobile and unable to close or to make a sound on closing. Thus, in severe calcific aortic stenosis, the aortic component of the second sound is generally "absent" and, since the aortic valve closure is the louder of the two components, there is an apparent "absence of the second sound" at the base (fig. 42). Similarly, in severe pulmonary valve stenosis, the pulmonary component of the second sound can hardly be heard owing to the involvement of its commissures and the low diastolic closing pressure transmitted from the pulmonary artery. The second sound at the base is, therefore, apparently single, only the aortic closure being heard. Alternatively, when one listens over the "pulmonary area" the aortic valve component may be lost in the pulmonary systolic murmur and with the faint closing sound of the pulmonary valve there is an apparent "absence of the second sound", as in aortic stenosis.

(b) The **varying interval between the components.** In normal circumstances there is a clinically detectable variation in the time interval between the two components of the second sound. On inspiration this gap widens and it narrows on expiration. This time variation should not be confused with the fact that the second sound is more clearly heard on expiration. The respiratory time variation results from an increased venous return from the systemic venous bed to the right heart.

In cases of atrial septal defect the splitting of the two components of the second sound is very wide and easily audible. This wide split of the second sound at the base is characteristic of atrial septal defect, but there is a further feature which is characteristic of the condition; the wide split does not vary appreciably with respiration. In other words, there is a wide "fixed" splitting of the second

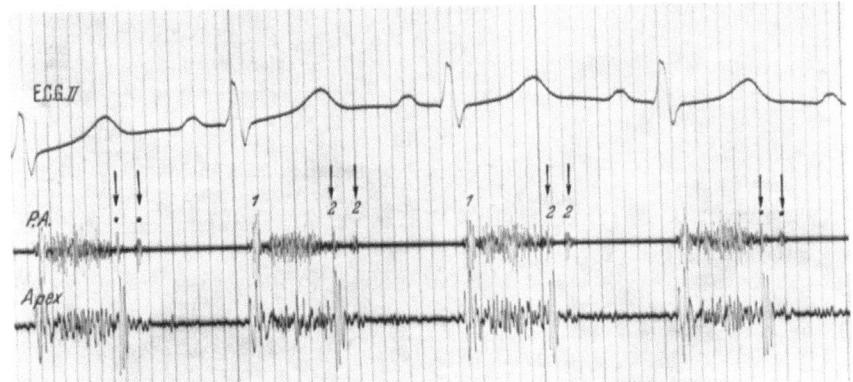

Fig. 44. In this case of atrial septal defect the two components of the second sound are widely spaced and "fixed", i.e. they do not vary with respiration

sound. The explanation of this phenomenon is not entirely clear at the present stage of our knowledge.

Where there is involvement of the left branch of the conducting bundle, there is delayed activation of the left ventricle, so that in certain circumstances aortic valve closure may actually come after pulmonary valve closure. Since the pulmonary component normally varies with respiration, we can, in these circumstances, have the two components narrowing with inspiration and widening with expiration, as the pulmonary component approaches and recedes from the markedly delayed aortic valve closure. Such a state of affairs is known as paradoxical or reversed splitting of the second sound. This generally requires confirmation from the phonocardiogram and electrocardiogram.

(c) **The loudness of the two components of the second sound.** The splitting of the second sound into two components indicates the presence of two functional valve units. But the loudness with which they close is an indication of the diastolic closing pressure in the aorta or pulmonary artery closing the valve leaflets. Thus, in essential hypertension with an aortic diastolic pressure of, say, 140 mm, there is a loud ringing closure of the aortic valve, best heard to the right of the sternum. In the evaluation of cardiac cases for surgery one is concerned with the presence of "pulmonary hypertension" so that we listen critically to the loudness of the pulmonary valve closure. This is best heard to the left of the sternum in the "pulmonary valve area". Where there is a high pulmonary artery pressure the pulmonary component of the second sound is loud and ringing. In the presence of collateral clinical evidence of pulmonary hypertension a loud pulmonary component of the second sound is helpful in confirming this feature. In severe pulmonary hypertension the shock of the pulmonary valve closure may be so marked as to be felt as an appreciable impulse with the flat of the hand held over the "pulmonary area" (p. 34).

The **Third Heart Sound** is of low-pitched intensity and is usually best heard at the "apex" of the heart. It is thought to represent a ventricular filling sound caused by the in-rush of blood into the ventricles in early diastole. One would, therefore, expect to hear it in cases with a large and dilated left ventricle such as occurs in left ventricular failure, mitral and aortic regurgitation.

The Fourth Heart Sound is due to atrial contraction and, therefore, immediately precedes the first heart sound and ventricular systole.

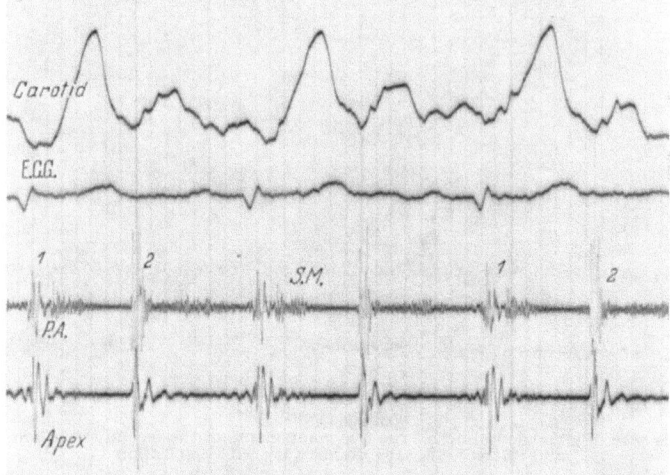

Fig. 45. This phonocardiogram is from a case of ventricular septal defect with pulmonary hypertension. The second sound at the pulmonary area is loud

Additional Sounds. In addition to the heart sounds already described, a number of extra sounds may be audible. The best known of these are the "opening snap" of the mitral valve and the pulmonary and aortic ejection sounds or clicks. These can all be conveniently regarded (for the purposes of surgical assessment), as representing "opening snaps" emanating from the mitral, pulmonary and aortic

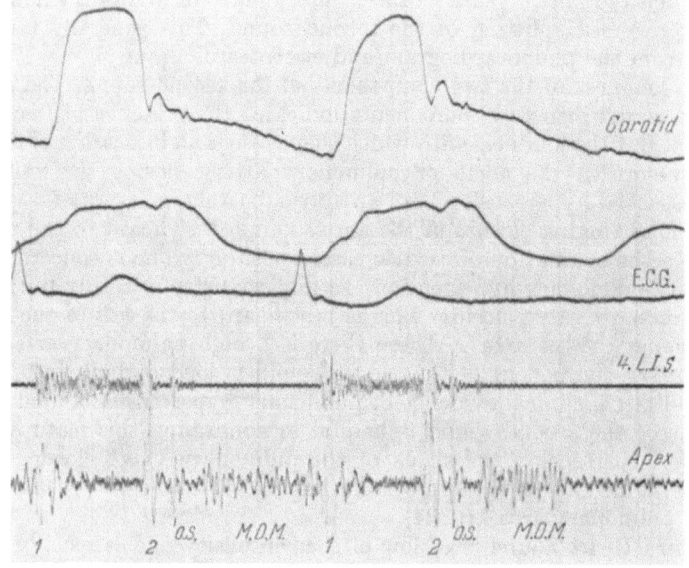

Fig. 46. The opening snap (O.S.) is most clearly audible medial to the apex. It follows the second sound and immediately precedes the mitral diastolic murmur (M.D.M.)

valves and their associated valve mechanisms. Although there is no general agreement on this point, their occurrence is, nevertheless, as a rule coincident with the time of opening of these valves.

The **opening snap of the mitral valve** suggests that the valve is abnormal and causes an audible sharp snapping sound as it opens; whereas the normal mitral valve gives rise to no opening sound. The presence of an opening snap (O. S.) usually indicates pliable mitral valve leaflets and, as such, is favourable from a surgical point of view. A heavily calcified valve rarely gives rise to an opening sound or, if present, it is indistinct. An opening sound is less common in mitral regurgitation but can be present with mobile valve leaflets. The opening snap of the mitral valve is best heard to the left of the sternum and just medial to the apex beat. Being related to mitral valve opening, it is heard just after the normal second sound, i. e. in early diastole and immediately before the rumbling diastolic murmur caused by the flow of blood through the valve (fig. 46).

It is high-pitched and may be mistaken for a late pulmonary component of the second sound. It is best heard towards the apex, while the pulmonary valve closure is heard most clearly at the "pulmonary area".

Aortic and pulmonary ejection sounds are heard just after the first sound and are coincident with the start of the systolic murmur caused by blood flow through the narrowed aortic or pulmonary valve. They are high pitched but may merge with the sound of the murmur. They are heard best about the fourth

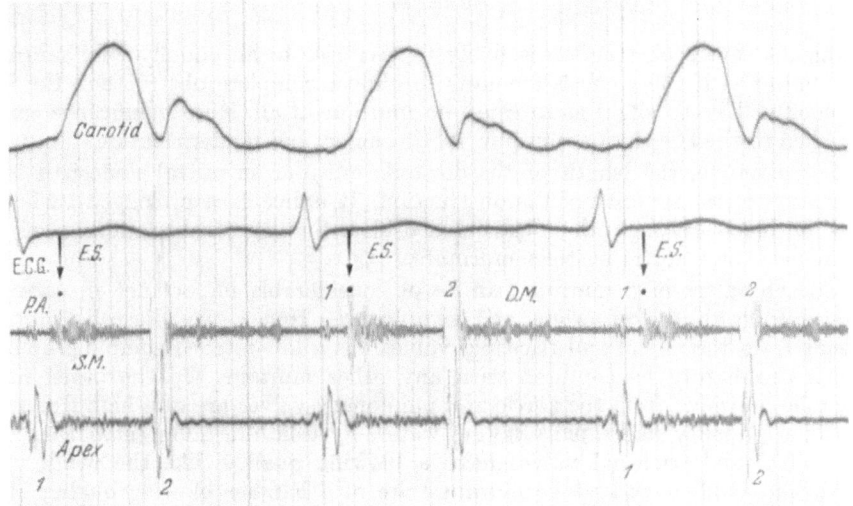

Fig. 47. In this case of persistent ductus arteriosus with pulmonary hypertension, an ejection sound (E.S.) can be distinguished coincident with the start of the systolic murmur at the pulmonary area. There is also a loud second sound and a diastolic murmur of pulmonary regurgitation

interspace to the left of the sternum or at the apex and the aortic ejection click may be heard up towards the root of the neck. Their presence is said to indicate a mild or moderate degree of stenosis of the valve and although the mechanism of their production is still under discussion, they could well represent opening snaps from these valves, the valve ring, or the adherent cusps. Just as the mitral opening snap may be mistaken for a split second sound, so aortic and pulmonary ejection sounds may resemble a split first sound.

Murmurs

These represent turbulence of the blood flow at such a frequency as to give rise to audible vibrations. It is unwise to attach undue significance to their interpretation. In particular, the loudness of a murmur does not necessarily indicate a severe lesion since a heavy flow of blood through an area of trivial obstruction gives rise to a loud murmur and, similarly, a small flow of blood

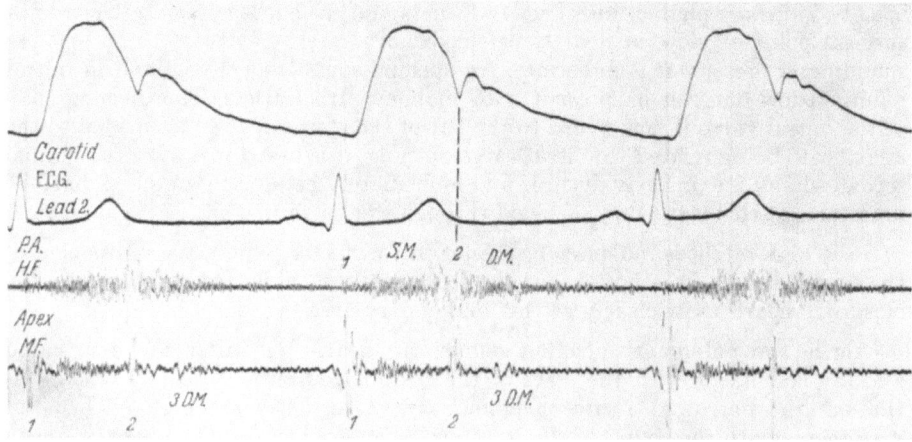

Fig. 48. The characteristic murmur of persistent ductus arteriosus which waxes in systole and wanes in diastole

through a severe obstruction is likely to give rise to an equally loud murmur. Alternatively, if the stenosis amounts to almost complete obstruction, the flow of blood will be so slight as to cause no murmur at all. More significance can be attached to the length of a murmur, its character, and its distribution.

For example, the **length** of the diastolic murmur in mitral stenosis is some indication of the severity of the obstruction. It indicates a prolonged turbulent flow of blood through the obstructed orifice. Similar considerations apply to pulmonary and aortic systolic murmurs.

The **character** of a murmur can be of considerable importance in correctly interpreting its site of origin and significance. Hence, the diastolic murmur arising from the mitral and tricuspid valves has a low-pitched rumbling quality, which can hardly be confused with any other murmur. On the other hand, diastolic murmurs from the aortic and pulmonary valves are of a high frequency "rushing" quality like rapidly falling water. Systolic murmurs emanating from the mitral and tricuspid valves have a blowing quality, like the wind, while aortic and pulmonary systolic murmurs are of a harsher blowing quality. It is easier to recognise the site of origin of a murmur by its character than by attempts to time it in relation to the cardiac cycle. This applies particularly where the heart rate is rapid.

The **distribution** of murmurs or their area of maximum intensity and direction of conduction can be helpful but better localisation can usually be gained from careful appraisal of associated thrills when present.

One should remember that murmurs are not confined to the immediate region of the heart. For example, the continuous murmur indicating a persistent ductus arteriosus may be heard most clearly below the left clavicle. Also, an arterio-venous communication elsewhere in the body will give rise to a similar continuous murmur. Also, an arterio-venous fistula of the lung, cirsoid aneurysm of the

In atrial septal defect it is usual to see a QRS pattern which is sometimes referred to as a "bundle branch block type" of pattern. This terminology is confusing, as the width of the complex is not increased and, as far as is known, there is no true block of the bundle branches.

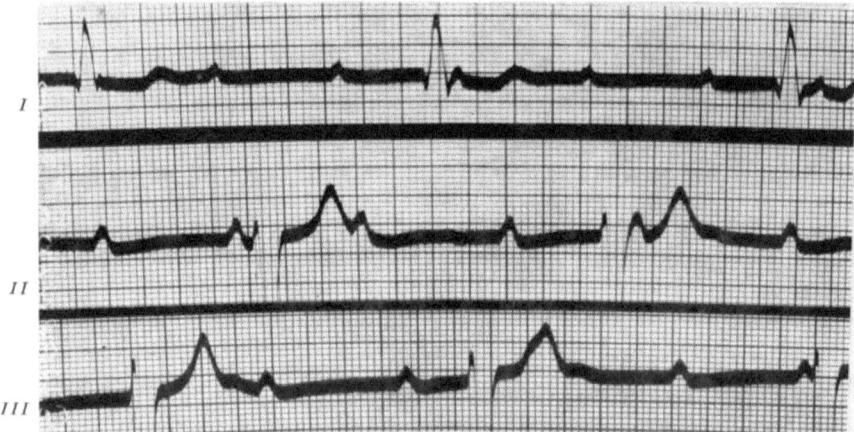

Fig. 66. Complete heart block. The P waves are unrelated to the ventricular complexes

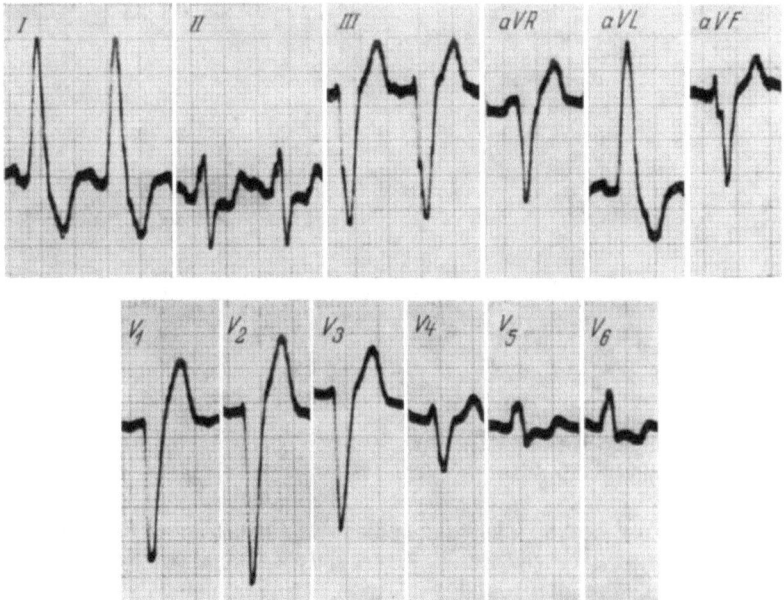

Fig. 67. Left bundle branch block. The ventricular complexes are widened and slurred

Ventricular tachycardia and **ventricular fibrillation** can be considered together. These abnormal rhythms are, unfortunately, quite common during cardiac surgery, particularly when dealing with diseased ventricles; for example, severe aortic stenosis. In ventricular tachycardia there is an abnormal area of excitability (ectopic focus) in the ventricle, giving rise to a rapid regular ventricular rhythm. The electrocardiographic picture should be familiar to all cardiac surgeons, since scalp, intra-cranial meningioma, or traumatic arteriovenous fistula in a limb all give rise to the same noise. Again, systolic murmurs may be heard over any area of vessel narrowing as, for example, in atheromatous narrowing of the aortic bifurcation and in the region of the carotid bifurcation.

In coarctation of the aorta, a systolic murmur may be heard posteriorly and to the left of the vertebral column at the site of the coarctation. Also in patients with a well-developed collateral bronchial circulation to the lungs (pulmonary atresia) the increased flow of blood in these vessels may give rise to a murmur, systolic or continuous, heard over the intercostal spaces posteriorly.

CHAPTER V

Special Investigations

In the routine investigation of a cardiological problem one should have information about the red cell count, the haemoglobin content of the blood, and the presence of abnormal constituents in the urine. In addition, a standard postero-anterior and left lateral view of the chest should be available, together with an electrocardiogram. These common-place investigations can scarcely be classified as being of a special nature; the term applies more particularly to right and left heart catheterization and angiocardiography.

An estimation of the haemoglobin content of the blood is valuable in all cases as a general index of the state of health of the patient. A falling haemoglobin may suggest the onset of bacterial endocarditis. In cyanotic congenital heart disease the haemoglobin content and degree of polycythaemia noted is an index of the severity of the disease. A reducing red cell count during the post-operative period can be a valuable guide to the adequacy of the surgical relief. Conversely, a rising haemoglobin is evidence of deterioration, particularly in FALLOT's tetralogy.

The urine will be examined as a routine in all cases of heart disease. Apart from abnormal constituents, a measurement of the volume of daily output serves as an indication of the response to treatment, particularly in cases of myocardial failure. The presence of microscopic haematuria may raise a suspicion of bacterial endocarditis.

Chest Radiography

This is an essential part of the examination and can reasonably be regarded as part of the "inspection" of the heart. A good postero-anterior chest radiograph can supply more useful objective information than the subjective impressions gained in a darkened room during fluoroscopy. In addition, a permanent record of the shape and size of the heart and the degree of vascularity of the lung fields is available for comparison at subsequent examinations.

On examining the chest film particular attention should be directed to

        (a) the bony cage
        (b) the cardiac outline (silhouette)
        (c) the lung fields.

(a) **The bony cage.** It is worth remembering that congenital anomalies frequently co-exist, so that it is not usual to find anomalies of the ribs or vertebral column in association with congenital heart disease. Hemivertebrae, with resulting scoliosis may occur, and supernumerary or bifid ribs are sometimes present. A

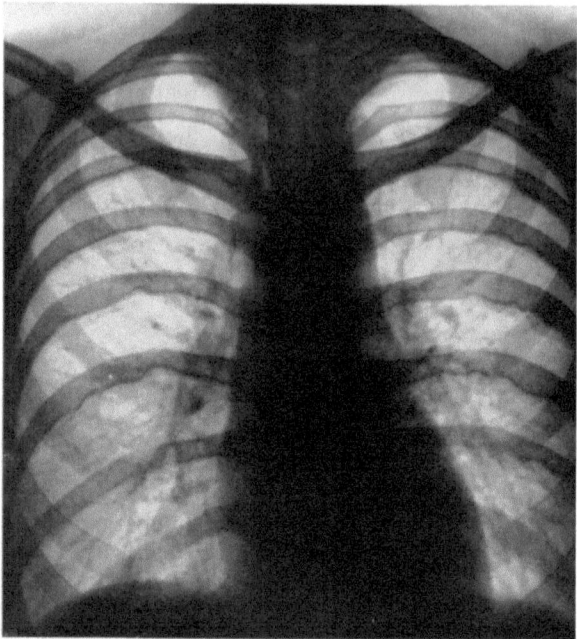

Fig. 49. A case of coarctation of the aorta showing well marked notching of the ribs

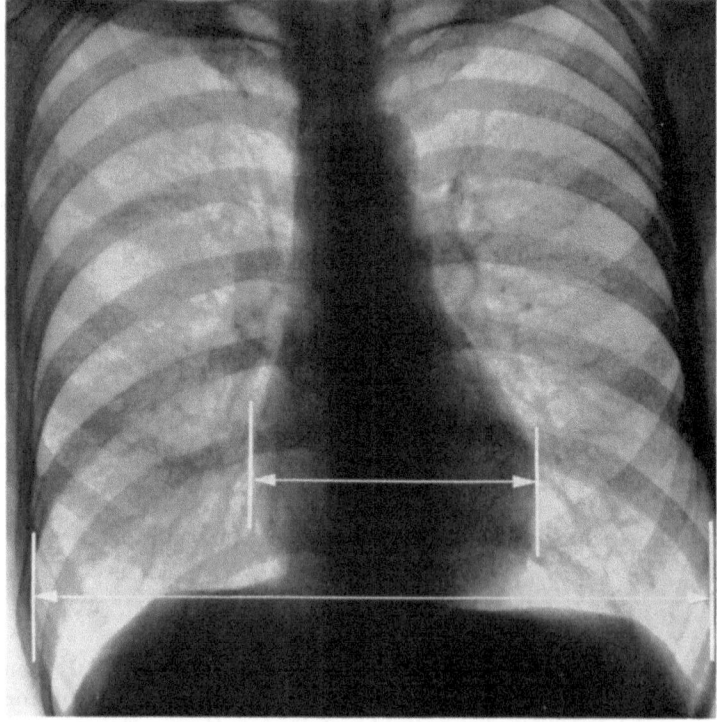

Fig. 50. The cardio-thoracic ratio is a measure of the transverse diameter of the heart and the greatest
width of the chest between the inner borders of the ribs

feature to look for is rib notching which, when bilateral, is virtually diagnostic of coarctation of the aorta. Unilateral rib notching is quite frequently seen after the Blalock operation, due to the development of a rich collateral arterial network supplying the arm on the side of the divided subclavian artery. Rib notching has also been described in severe cyanotic heart disease, like pulmonary atresia, where the collateral blood supply to the lungs is heavy. Erosion of the ribs may be seen in aneurysm.

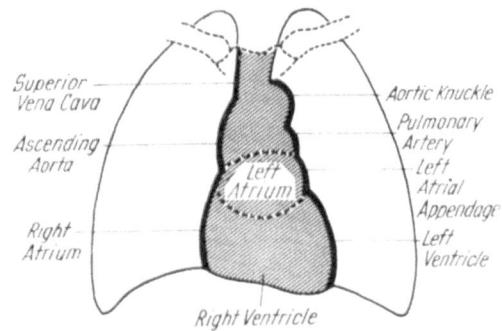

Fig. 51. An interpretation of the bulges on the cardiac shadow as seen in the standard postero-anterior chest radiograph

(b) **The cardiac outline.** It is possible to gain an impression of an increase in the bulk of the cardiac shadow from casual inspection. In obstructive lesions the muscular hypertrophy is initially concentric, with little increase in the size of the heart. A large heart favours conditions associated with a large stroke volume, like aortic regurgitation, mitral regurgitation, or a septal defect. Where it develops rapidly in the presence of a stenotic lesion, it suggests myocardial failure and dilatation. A postoperative increase in the size of the heart shadow may be due to a number of these factors but it is equally likely to be the result of an accumulation of pericardial fluid. The size of the heart is conveniently measured and expressed as the *cardio-thoracic ratio*. This is normally under 50 per cent and the measurement should be entered in the patient's notes at each examination.

Localised areas of hypertrophy or dilatation of the

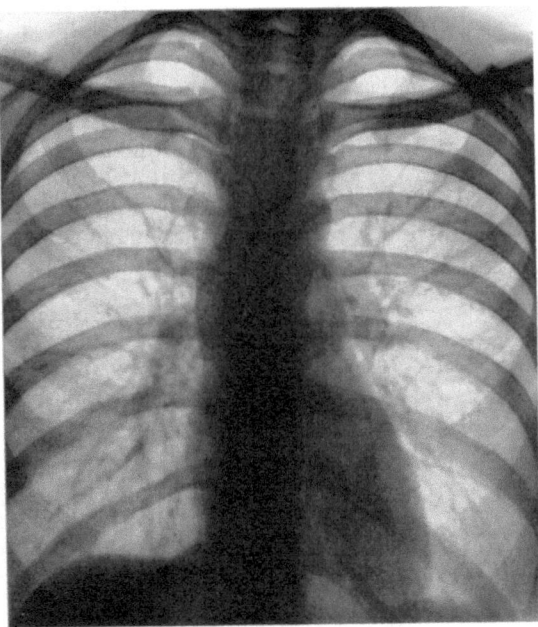

Fig. 52. The post-stenotic bulge of the ascending aorta is well seen in aortic valve stenosis

cardiac silhouette can be of great diagnostic value, so that it is essential to have a clear image of what constitutes the normal outline when viewed in the postero-anterior projection. This is best indicated in the accompanying drawings (fig. 51).

It will be appreciated that these contours will not be visible on all cardiac outlines, but where a localised projection occurs its underlying cause can often be inferred from a mind's-eye anatomical concept of the position of the heart within the chest.

The **superior caval** shadow is not of great diagnostic value but the corresponding shadow of the left side may indicate the presence of a left superior vena cava.

Again, an aortic arch descending on the right side (present in 25% of FALLOT's tetralogy) may make the normal superior caval shadow appear unduly prominent.

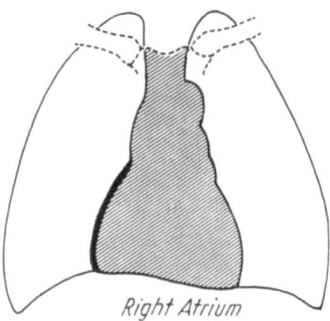

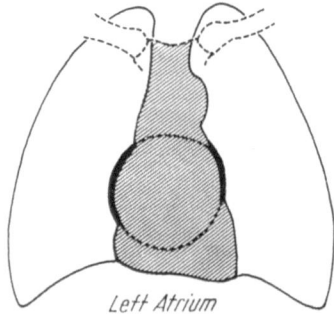

Fig. 53. The features of right and left atrial enlargement as seen in the chest radiograph

The **aortic arch** is visible in two areas on the postero-anterior projection — in its ascending part above the valve and as the "aortic knuckle" on the left border.

A prominent ascending aorta is the rule in aortic valve stenosis and represents one example of post-stenotic dilatation (see p. 13). It should be looked for in every case of aortic stenosis and where absent should make one reconsider the diagnosis or suspect the possibility of a sub-valvar obstruction. In conditions of atherosclerotic unfolding of the aorta, syphilitic aortic regurgitation, or the dilated aorta of essential hypertension, the ascending aorta will again be prominent, but the rest of the aorta, including the "knuckle" should be equally prominent (fig. 52).

The size of the aortic knuckle is a good indication of the size of the aorta and also indicates whether the arch is right-sided or descends in its normal position on the left. In the presence of a left-to-right-shunt, a small aortic knuckle favours a diagnosis of atrial septal defect or ventricular septal defect, while a large knuckle is in favour of a persistent ductus arteriosus. This can be a useful differential feature. In general terms, a small aorta suggests a small cardiac

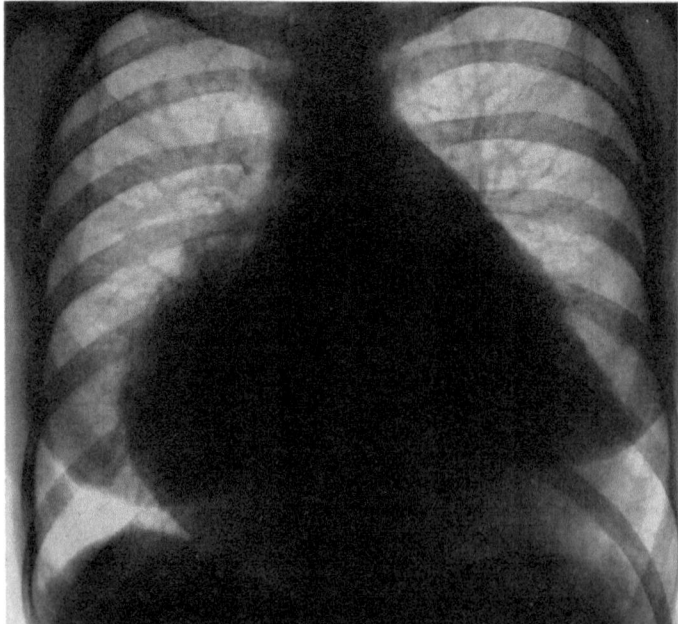

Fig. 54. A grossly enlarged left atrium in a case of mitral valve disease. The left atrial shadow projects on both cardiac borders

output in cases with an obstructive lesion and, conversely, a normal sized aorta suggests a mild or moderate obstruction and a normal cardiac output.

In coarctation of the aorta there may be an "absent" aortic knuckle, with a prominent left subclavian artery or alternatively, a "double aortic knuckle" caused by overlapping shadows of the left subclavian artery and the post-stenotic dilatation of the descending aorta below the coarctation.

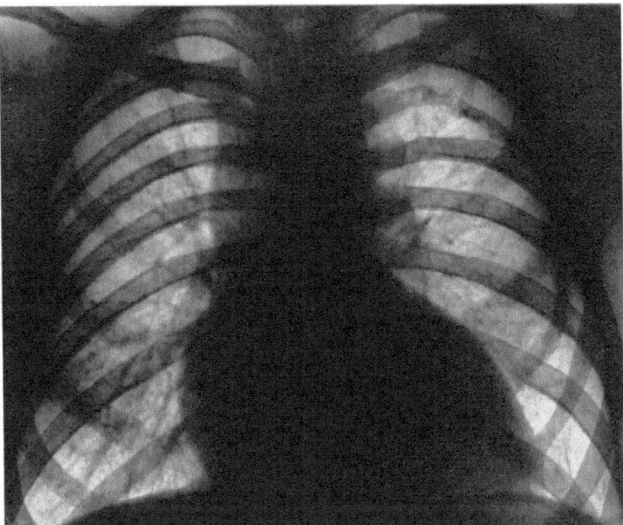

Fig. 55. An enlarged left ventricle in a case of aortic regurgitation

Enlargement of the right and left atria may indicate either stenosis or regurgitation at the tricuspid or mitral valves respectively. Right atrial enlargement shows as a ballooning of the lower right border of the heart, extending down to the diaphragm and blunting the right cardio-phrenic angle. Left atrial enlargement is seen as a globular shadow of increased density within the cardiac silhouette (characteristically in mitral stenosis).

Very considerable enlargement — sometimes called aneurysmal dilatation of the left atrium — protrudes beyond both cardiac borders and may tend to be confused with the right atrial enlargement. The lower border adjacent to the right cardio-phrenic angle, tends in these cases to swing sharply inwards, forming an acute cardio-phrenic angle, as opposed to the blunt angle of right atrial enlargement. In addition, the convexity of the left atrium or the left atrial appendage on the left border of the heart shadow tends to be unduly prominent. Aneurysmal dilatation of the left atrium in the presence of mitral valve disease favours a diagnosis of mitral regurgitation.

The Ventricles. It is worth re-emphasizing that there can be considerable concentric hypertrophy of the obstructed right or left ventricle without evidence of enlargement of the ventricular silhouette. Where these chambers are grossly hypertrophied or dilated, they have a characteristic contour. The right ventricle is adjacent to the central tendon of the diaphragm, and enlargement of this chamber tends to elevate the heart and "round off" the apex. Sometimes this contour is obscured by the diaphragm or can be seen through the stomach gas bubble.

With left ventricular hypertrophy the left ventricle, which constitutes the normal left lower border of the cardiac shadow, enlarges outwards and downwards

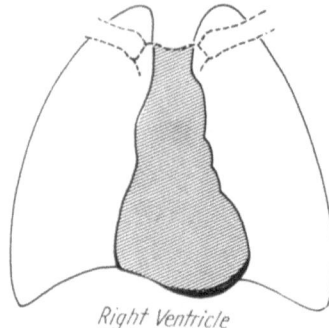

Right Ventricle

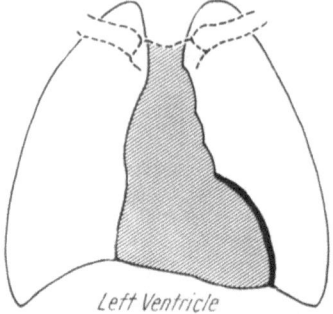

Left Ventricle

Fig. 56. Diagram emphasising the features of right and left ventricular enlargement

towards the diaphragm, producing a "sharp apex" unlike the elevated round apex of right ventricular enlargement.

The Lateral Chest Radiograph. A true lateral picture should always be available, since it is only with the aid of a postero-anterior and lateral projection that any doubtful opacity of the lungs or abnormal cardiac shadow can be accurately located within the chest.

In addition, the lateral projection is of value in demonstrating calcification of the valve cusps. Particularly in aortic stenosis, the demonstration of calcification of the valve leaflets indicates that the stenosis is at valve level and not subvalvar. A suspicion of valve calcification can often be confirmed by fluoroscopy, tomography, or oblique projections. The calcified aortic valve lies well within the substance of the cardiac shadow. Calcification of the pericardium also shows up to advantage on a lateral chest radiograph.

The interpretation of oblique views of the cardiac contour falls more within the field of the radiologist and physician cardiologist, as do oesophagograms, which delineate the aortic and cardiac contours adjacent to the barium-filled oesophagus. The aortic indentation of the oesophagus can be of help in determining the size of the aorta and the side on which it descends. Also, some cases of double aortic arch can be demonstrated in this way. Enlargement of the left atrium distorts the oesophagus backwards in a sickle-shaped curve.

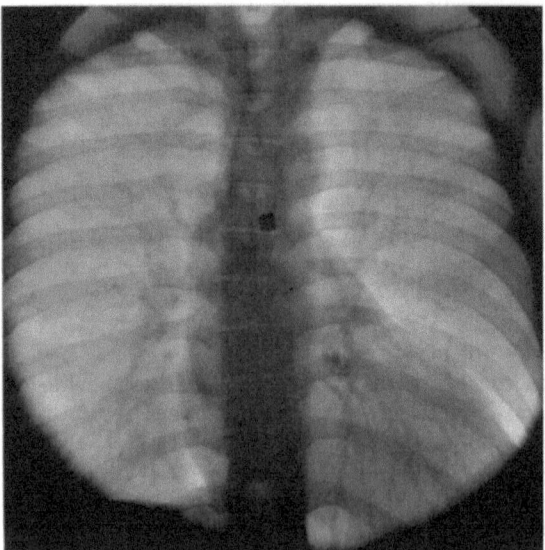

a

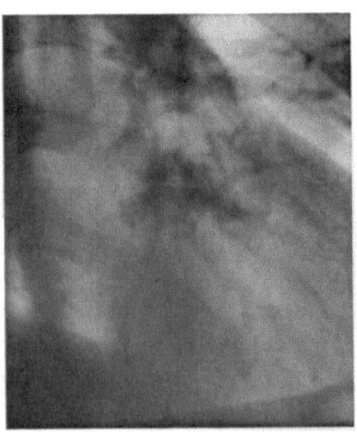

b

Fig. 57 a and b. (P.A. and Lateral) Calcification of the aortic valve

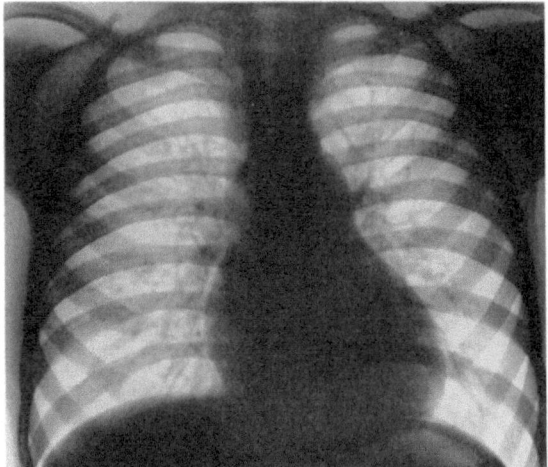

Fig. 58. Oligaemic lung fields in pulmonary stenosis. Note the post-stenotic bulge of the pulmonary artery

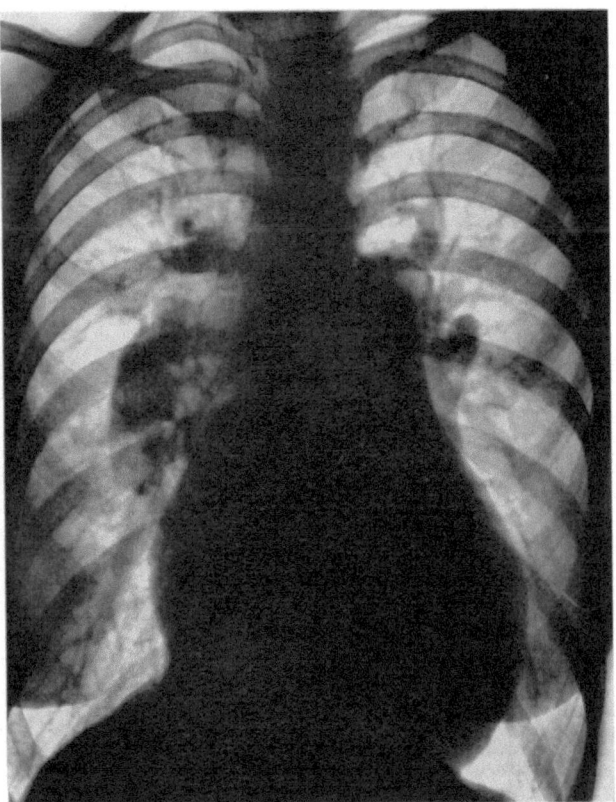

Fig. 59. The lung fields in pulmonary hypertension with reversed shunt through a ventricular septal
defect. The outer one-third of the lung fields is clear

(c) **The Lung Fields.** Examination of these is important in any cardiac con
dition, chiefly from the point of view of the degree of vascularity of the lungs.
Other features, like pleural effusions, and haemosiderosis should also be noted.

Reduced vascularity of the lung fields occurs in pulmonary stenosis presenting either as an isolated lesion or as part of FALLOT's tetralogy. In the former condition there may be a prominent pulmonary arterial trunk proximally (post-stenotic

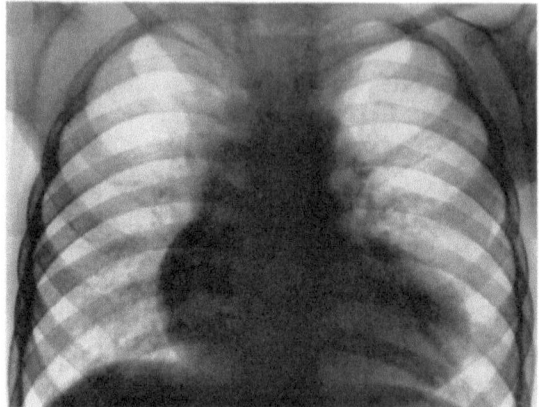

Fig. 60. In severe pulmonary stenosis or pulmonary atresia the bronchial vascular pattern predominates as a uniform shadowing with poor main pulmonary vessels

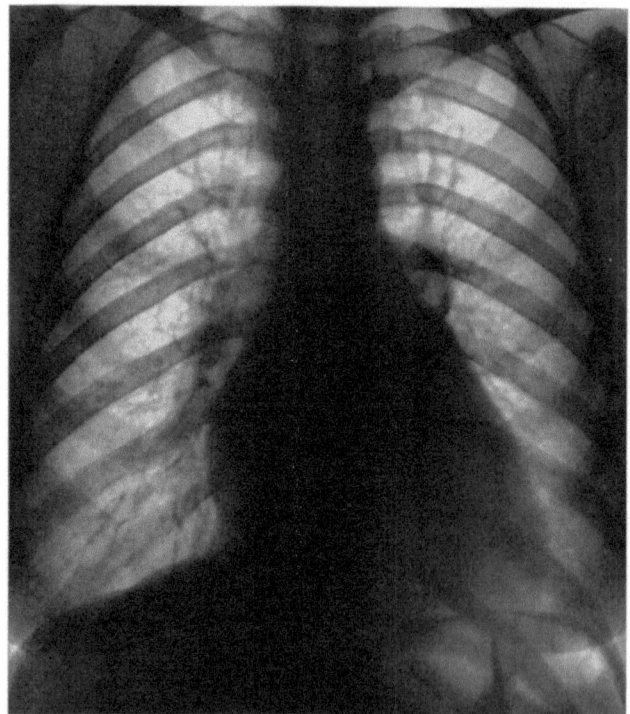

Fig. 61. Congestion of the lungs associated with mitral stenosis (passive congestion). Short horizontal basal lines in the costo-phrenic angles known as Kerleylines are not seen at this magnification

dilatation, p. 13), but the vascular shadows of the vessels diminish rapidly and at the periphery the lung fields are "clear". This picture should not be confused with that seen in severe pulmonary hypertension. Here, only the peripheral subdivisions of the vascular tree are affected, producing a clear lung field in the outer zones, but the hila and middle zones of the lung are occupied by prominent and enlarged pulmonary arteries. This picture is well seen in the Eisenmenger group of conditions.

Lungs with a diminished vascular pattern are known as *oligaemic* lung fields.

In some severe cases of pulmonary stenosis or pulmonary atresia, the lung fields are superficially not oligaemic, but appear to be uniformly and diffusely

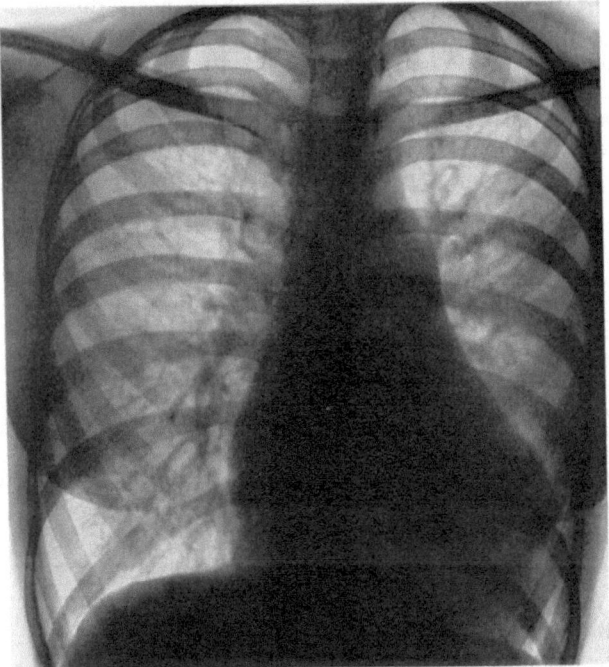

Fig. 62. Hyperaemic lung fields indicating a heavy left-to-right shunt in atrial septal defect. Note the right atrial and pulmonary artery enlargements

mottled with small vascular shadows — an appearance somewhat resembling miliary tuberculosis. On close inspection, the proximal pulmonary arterial trunks are absent, rudimentary, or spidery in pattern. The diffuse uniform mottling is thought to be due to extensive bronchial artery-pulmonary artery anastomoses which maintain the pulmonary circulation (fig. 60).

Where there is an increased vascularity of the lungs, one should try to distinguish between cases of "passive congestion" associated with mitral stenosis or left ventricular failure and the actively congested lungs typical of left-to-right shunts. The former condition affects chiefly the veins and is more noticeable in the dependent lobes. There may be associated collections of pleural fluid and an important corroborative feature is the presence of KERLEY's lines.

KERLEY's lines are short horizontal lines about 1 to 1.5 cm long most clearly seen in the costophrenic angles. They occur in association with an increased pulmonary venous pressure. They are most often seen in cases of mitral stenosis with congestive features and in any case with features of pulmonary oedema or paroxysmal nocturnal dyspnoea.

Active congestion of the lungs is known as pulmonary plethora and the lung fields are then described as *pleonaemic*. This is due to a great increase of blood flow through the pulmonary bed and there is a gross uniform increase of vascularity and general vascular shadowing involving the arteries and the veins. Pulmonary plethora occurs particularly in atrial septal defect, ductus arteriosus, ventricular septal defect, or any other condition with a considerable left-to-right shunt.

The Electrocardiograph

The interpretation of the electrocardiograph in heart disease has become a complex study and, for the finer shades of interpretation, one's cardiological colleague should be consulted. It is, however, important for the cardiac surgeon to have some rudimentary concept of the electrocardiographic pattern in order to be able to add to or to confirm his clinical impression.

It is customary to have recordings of the three standard limb leads, three unipolar limb leads, and six V leads, or unipolar praecordial leads.

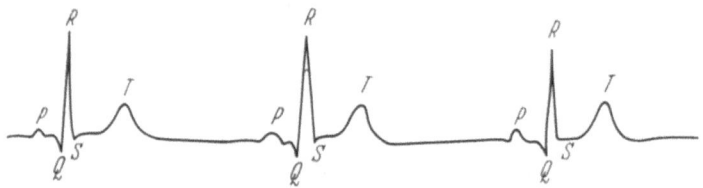

Fig. 63. The normally seen electrical deflections of the electrocardiograph "U". Waves are small positive deflections following the T which are sometimes accentuated by digitalis

It should be emphasized that the electrocardiograph in no way represents the cardiac impulse or the pressure changes within the ventricles. It is simply a recording of the electrical impulses or disturbances which pass through the cardiac muscle mass, and precede the actual mechanical events.

The wave pattern produced is basically similar in all instances; the various identifiable components being known by the letters P, Q, R, S, T.

The P wave represents the passage of the impulse through the atria. The time interval between the P wave and the beginning of the Q, R, S, T, complex of waves is the P. R. interval and represents the passage of the impulse through the av node, bundle of His and its branches. The Q R S complex of waves is produced by the electrical depolarisation spreading through both ventricles, while the T wave is thought to represent repolarisation or re-establishment of the charge or membrane potential on the muscle.

The electrocardiograph can be of help to the cardiac surgeon in confirming or interpreting disturbances of rhythm and in establishing hypertrophy of one or more chambers of the heart.

Disturbance of Rhythm

The commonest arrhythmia encountered in surgical practice is *atrial fibrillation*. It is usual in cases of rheumatic mitral stenosis and commonly occurs post-operatively in this condition if not present before operation. Less frequently it complicates atrial septal defect. The presence of atrial fibrillation in association with isolated aortic stenosis should make one consider a rheumatic aetiology for this condition and an associated involvement of the mitral valve.

Clinically, there is total irregularity of the volume and rate of the pulse. The condition may be confused with multiple extrasystoles or atrial flutter with changing atrio-ventricular block. The electrocardiograph is, however, characteristic with absence of P waves and a varying distance between the ventricular complexes.

A regularly recurring irregularity, every second beat being premature and followed by a compensatory pause, is known as *pulsus bigeminus*. It may indicate digitalis intoxication. The electrocardiograph reveals this as a normal beat followed by an ectopic beat (p. 26).

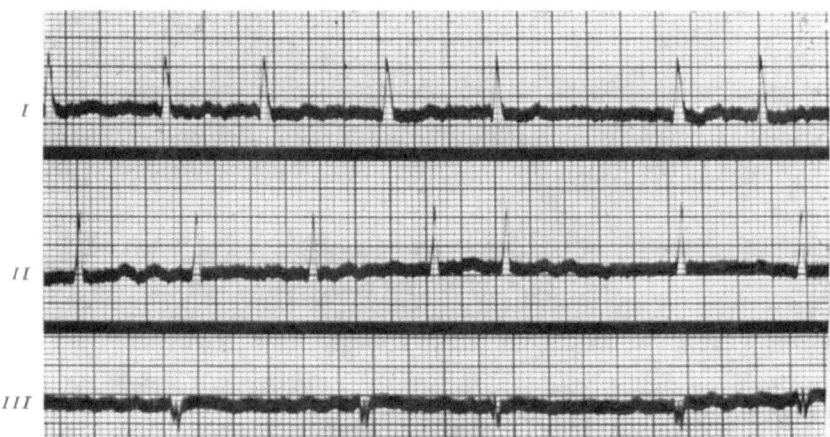

Fig. 64. Atrial fibrillation. The P waves are absent and the QRS complexes are irregularly spaced

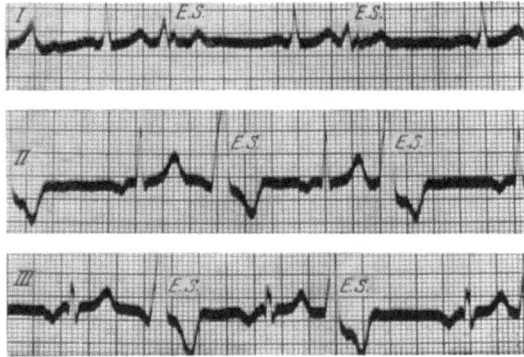

Fig. 65. Pulsus bigeminus-each normal complex is followed by an extrasystole (ES.)

The cardiac surgeon should be alive to the various types and significance of persistent post-operative tachycardias, for management will depend upon a precise diagnosis.

Abnormally slow heart rates may indicate a condition of *heart block*. Since the advent of surgery for ventricular septal defect, traumatic heart block is not uncommon. Here, the atria and ventricles are dissociated and beat at their own independent rhythm — the ventricular rate, indicated by the QRST, being much slower than the atrial (P wave) rate. The PR interval is, of course, quite inconstant (fig. 66).

Where the conduction of the impulse through the branches of the bundle is impaired or interrupted, the co-ordinated and synchronised electrical activity in the right and left ventricles which produce the QRS complex will be disturbed. There is then usually widening and a bizarre or splintered QRS pattern. This is known as bundle branch block (fig. 67).

it is likely to proceed to ventricular fibrillation if the abnormal focus cannot be controlled.

Ventricular fibrillation probably results from a series of ectopic foci within the ventricular muscle mass, with large segments of the ventricle contracting independently. Such a rhythm cannot produce a co-ordinated ventricular contraction and, if untreated, is invariably fatal.

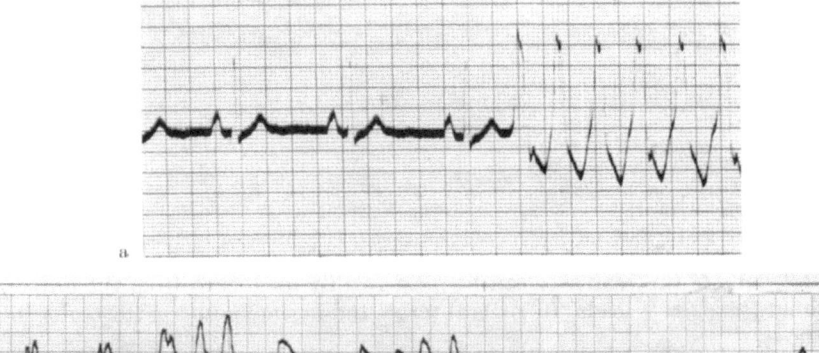

Fig. 68. a The onset of ventricular tachycardia. b Ventricular fibrillation

Cardiac Hypertrophy

Hypertrophy of the atria may involve the right or left atrium and the changes are reflected in the P wave. Left atrial hypertrophy, which is characteristic of mitral stenosis, produces a widened, flattened and bifid P wave. This is often best

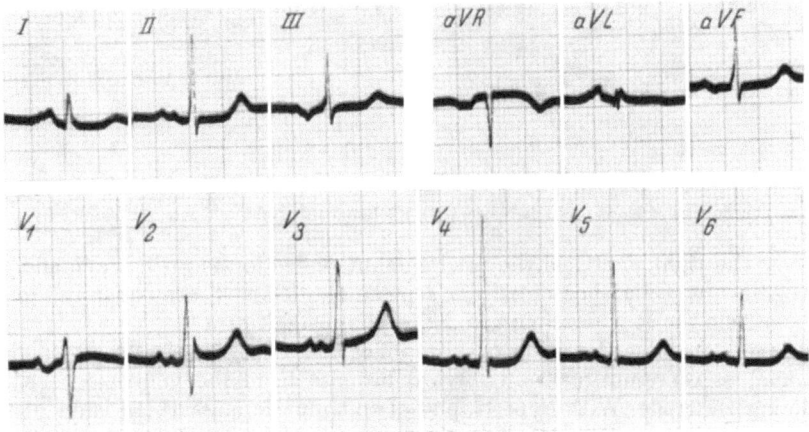

Fig. 69. P Mitrale. The wave is broad and with a double deflection

seen in standard limb lead II and is known as the "P mitrale". Right atrial hypertrophy is revealed as a high spiked P wave, sometimes known as the "P pulmonale". It may be present in any condition causing increased right atrial pressure e. g. pulmonary valve stenosis.

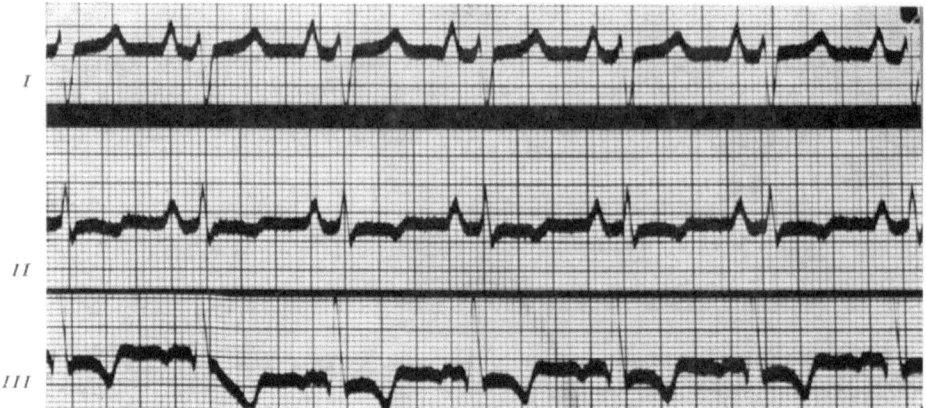

Fig. 70. The high spiked P waves of right atrial hypertrophy. The three standard limb leads are shown

Hypertrophy of the ventricles can be most readily diagnosed from the unipolar praecordial leads, or V leads. In general terms the normal adult pattern obtained is as follows:

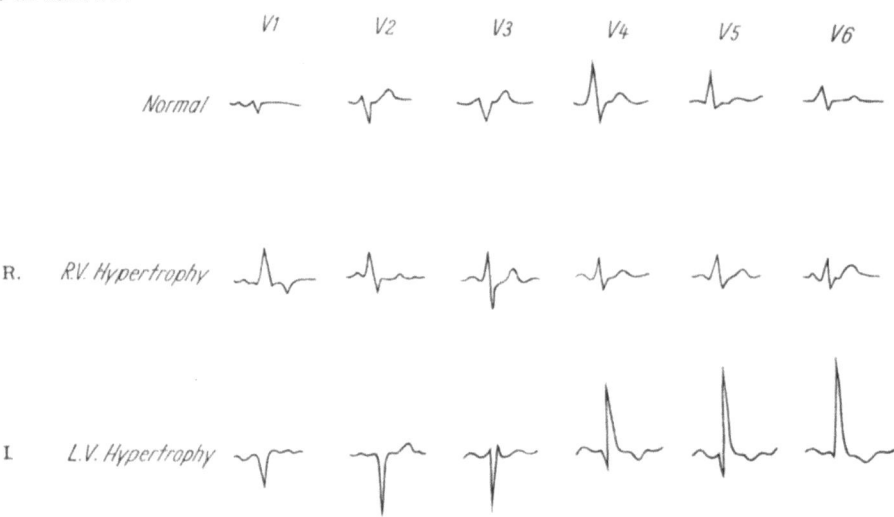

Fig. 71. The normal V leads and the characteristic changes of right and left ventricular hypertrophy

Over the right ventricle the predominant deflection is an S wave and the R is insignificant. Over the ventricular septum the R and S are equal and over the left ventricle the R is dominant and the S is insignificant.

It is convenient, although an oversimplification, to regard the positive deflection (R wave) as representing the electrical impulse from the ventricle beneath the exploring electrode. With hypertrophy of this muscle mass there is an increased amplitude of the positive electrical wave pattern.

Therefore, in right ventricular hypertrophy the positive wave or R wave should be increased in the leads taken over that ventricle, i.e. increased R waves in say V 1, 2, and 3. In left ventricular hypertrophy there is corresponding increase in the positive electrical deflection (R wave) over the left ventricular leads, i.e. V4, 5, and 6.

As the left ventricle is normally thicker than the right ventricle, the deflections from that ventricle dominate the normal electrocardiographic picture.

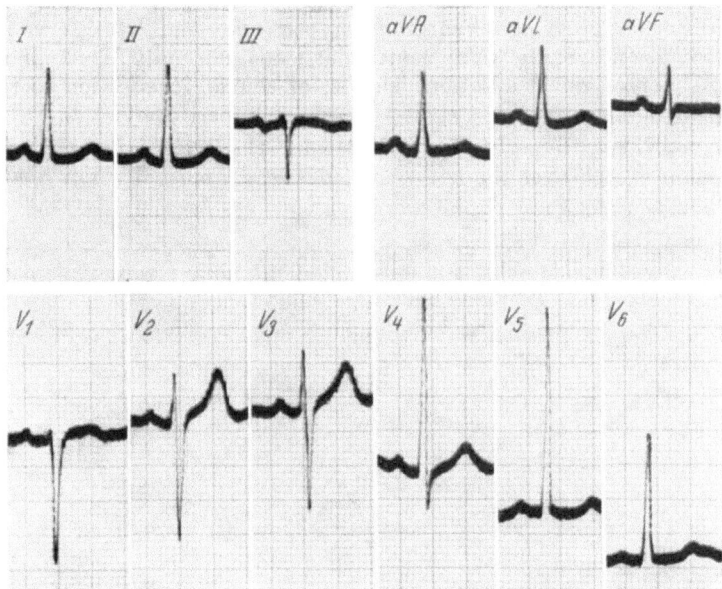

Fig. 72. The picture of left ventricular hypertrophy with big positive deflections over V 4, 5 and 6

"Strain" Patterns

In cases of severe ventricular hypertrophy it is usual to see an inversion of the T wave over the distribution of the ventricle in "strain". Where this is marked, the T is not only inverted but the ST segment may also be depressed below the iso-electric level.

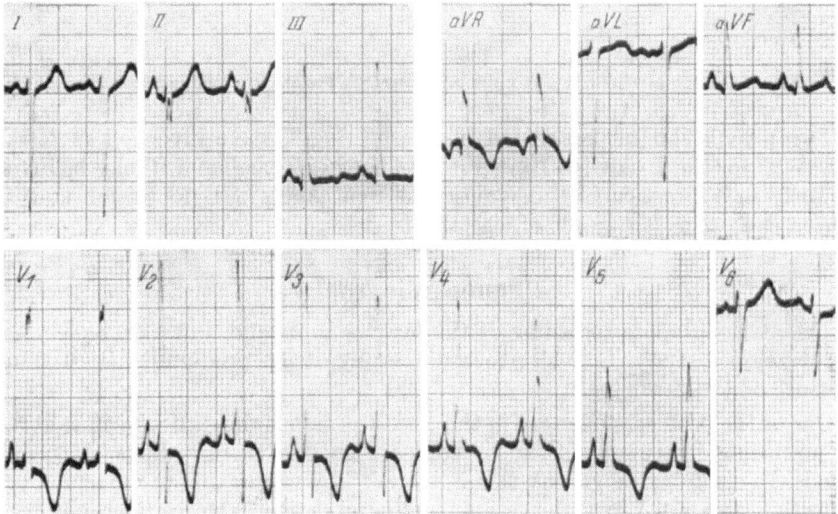

Fig. 73. Right ventricular hypertrophy and strain. Note the big positive deflections in V1—4 and the deeply inverted T waves

The cause of these deflections is not known with certainty but they resemble the patterns seen in ischaemic heart disease, and it is reasonable to assume that the grossly hypertrophied underlying muscle is, in fact, out-stripping its blood supply.

In conditions of gross right ventricular hypertrophy and "strain" we therefore expect T inversion over the right ventricular leads, normally V1, 2, and 3, with possibly ST depression in addition. This is, of course, in addition to the other electrocardiographic features of right ventricular hypertrophy.

In left ventricular hypertrophy and "strain" the T inversion and sometimes ST depression is seen over the left ventricular leads, normally V4, 5, and 6.

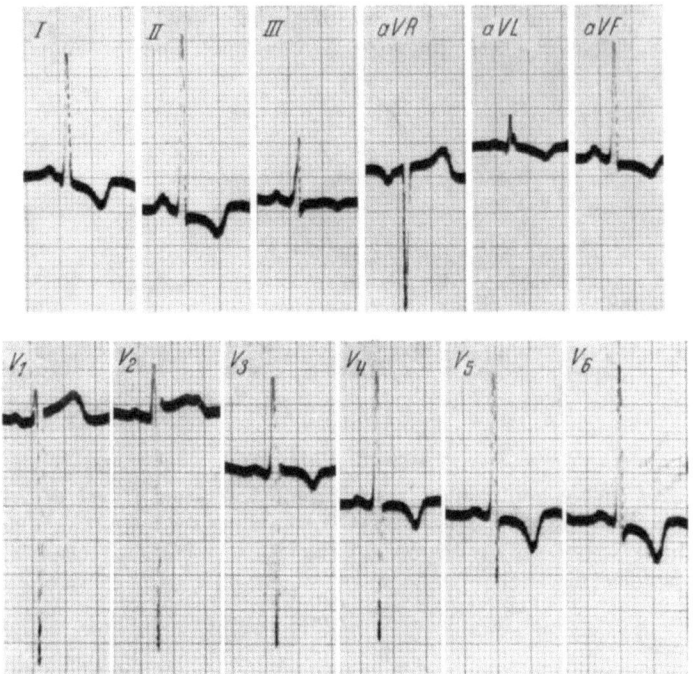

Fig. 74. Left ventricular hypertrophy and "strain". T wave inversion is seen in V 3—6

Two pitfalls should be avoided in interpreting T wave inversion as "strain". It is usual for the T wave to be inverted in V1 in all cases and it may be inverted normally in V2 or even V3 in young children. Again, ST depression and T inversion can occur as a result of digitalis.

Phonocardiography

This is the graphic recording of the heart sounds and murmurs and is now a well-developed study. Like electrocardiography, it lies predominantly within the province of the cardiologist.

One of the problems inherent in this investigation is the difficulty in calibrating the recording instrument so as to compare successive recordings of the heart sounds. In electrocardiography this is achieved by calibrating the machine before use with a standard 1 m.v. deflection; furthermore, in electrocardiography records are taken from well established standard positions on the chest wall. The heart sounds on the other hand are generally recorded in the area in which they are best heard. The chief value of the instrument lies in the accurate timing of the heart sounds, murmurs, and additional sounds in relation to one another, and to other events in the cardiac cycle.

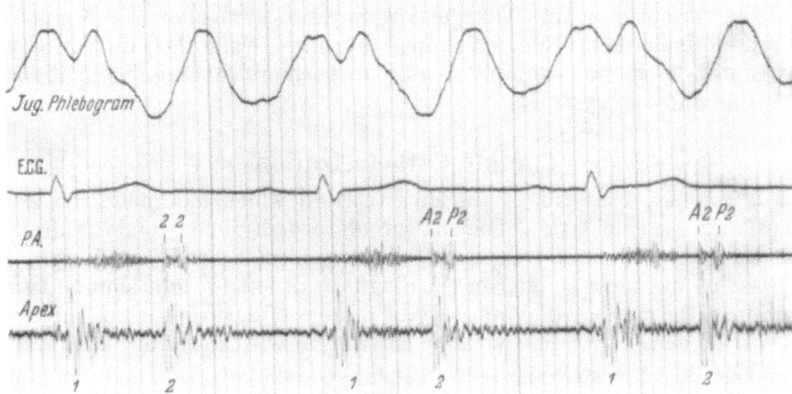

Fig. 75. The phonocardiogram relates the heart sounds to other events in the cardiac cycle. In this tracing the two components of the second sound are clearly indicated

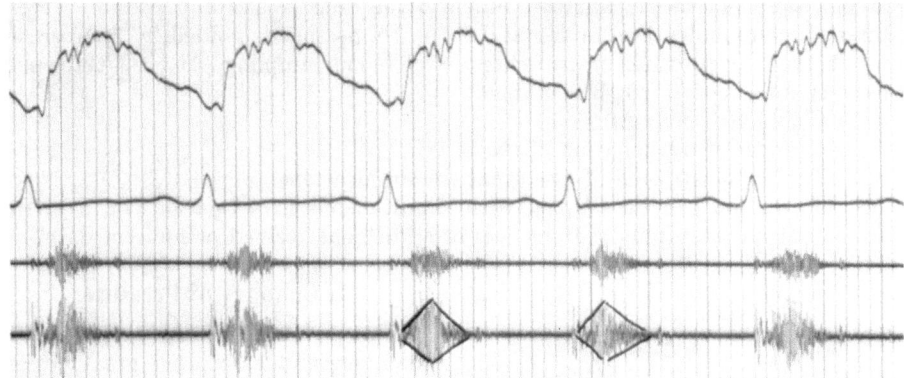

Fig. 76. An obstructive systolic murmur from a case of aortic stenosis. The murmur has a diamond shape and follows the first sound

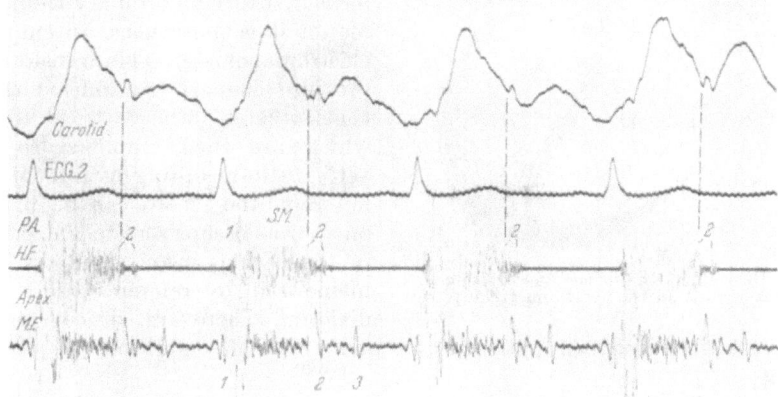

Fig. 77. The systolic murmur of ventricular septal defect. The murmur is coincident with the first sound and occupies the whole of systole

In addition, some information may be obtained from a study of the recorded shape of the various murmurs. Obstructive murmurs at the aortic and pulmonary valves produce spindle or diamond shaped murmurs, while the murmur of a ventricular septal defect, for example, is said to be more rectangular in shape and occupies the whole of systole.

Cardiac Catheterization

It is fair to say that this is the investigation which has made the greatest contribution to the elucidation of normal circulatory physiology and the alterations brought about by disease. In general, in congenital heart disease, right heart catheterization has most to offer in the diagnosis of left-to-right shunts. In right-to-left shunts, the angiocardiogram may be more useful, since the opaque medium is then carried across into the systemic circulation with the shunt stream.

The newer associated techniques of left heart catheterization and dye injection studies have added greatly to the information obtainable at cardiac catheterization.

Right heart catheterization involves the passage of a radio-opaque catheter through the right heart chambers out into the lung vessels and possibly across abnormal communications or septal defects. Its passage is guided by fluoroscopy and checked by pressure measurements and blood sampling. At least three sets of direct information can be obtained.

(1) Changes of pressure
(2) Changes of oxygenation of the blood
(3) The demonstration of abnormal communications.

This information can be coupled with simultaneous investigations of, say, the cardiac output, to supply a great deal of additional derived or indirect data.

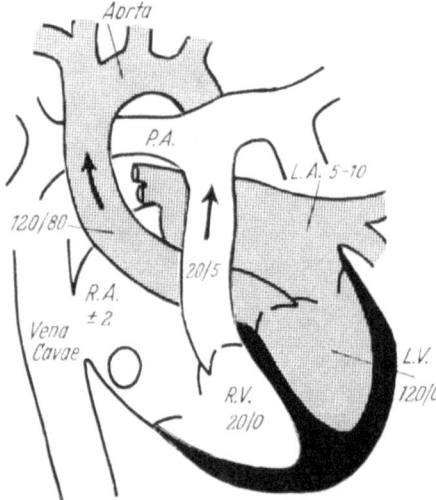

Fig. 78. Diagram indicating the approximate normal pressures within the heart and great vessels

1. Changes of Pressure

The pressures within various heart chambers and associated great vessels are usually express in mm. Hg. above an arbitrary zero level or base line, from which the recording instrument is calibrated. Although pressures have been measured with an ordinary saline manometer, it is more usual to employ an electromanometer. This transforms the pressure changes transmitted through the catheter into electrical impulses which are then amplified so as to activate the recording instrument. Alternatively, the record can be projected on an oscilloscope screen. The pressures in the various heart chambers can be memorised by reference to a simple diagram. There are, of course, fairly wide variations between patients and under various conditions in the same patient.

The pressure in the right atrium and great veins is low and reflects the low intra-thoracic pressure which, in some phases of respiration is negative. a, c, and v waves (p. 30) are distinguishable in the right atrial record. The right ventricular systolic pressure is generally between 20 and 30 mm. Hg. with a zero diastolic pressure. Where the diastolic pressure is raised it may indicate pulmonary regurgitation or a failing right ventricle. The systolic pressure in the pulmonary artery will be the same as that in the right ventricle provided there is no obstruction (functional or organic) at the pulmonary valve or in the right ventricular outflow. There is, however, a positive diastolic pressure in the pulmonary artery. This results from pulmonary valve closure as the right ventricular pressure falls. The normal systolic/diastolic pulmonary artery pressure is in the region of 25/10 mm. As with aortic regurgitation, pulmonary regurgitation is usually revealed by a wide pulmonary artery pulse pressure with a raised systolic and low diastolic pressure.

In the course of the blood flow through the smaller pulmonary arteries and arterioles, there is a progressive fall in pressure so that in the pulmonary capillaries and the pulmonary veins beyond, the pressure has fallen to 5—10 mm. Hg. This is the pressure generally recorded in the left atrium (this left atrial pressure being generated by the right ventricle, p. 14). Measurement of this left atrial pressure can be obtained at right heart catheterization by wedging the cardiac catheter in a distal pulmonary artery branch, so as to block the vessel completely. The pressure then recorded is known as the **pulmonary capillary venous** (P.C.V.) or **wedge-pressure,** and represents the pressure distal to the blocking catheter, i. e. the left atrial pressure.

The accuracy of the pulmonary capillary wedge pressure in reflecting the true left atrial pressure has been verified on a number of occasions by comparing the pressure obtained with that recorded by direct left atrial needle puncture. The left atrial pressure tracing shows the same a, c, v positive deflections and x, y negative deflections as can be recorded from the right atrium.

Measurements of pressures obtained at cardiac catheterization are particularly useful in diagnosing obstructive lesions especially at the level of the pulmonary valve or the infundibulum of the right ventricle. They are also of use in diagnosing tricuspid stenosis and through the pulmonary capillary wedge pressure we have an indication of the left atrial pressure. From this it is possible to estimate the degree of any existing mitral stenosis. Straightforward

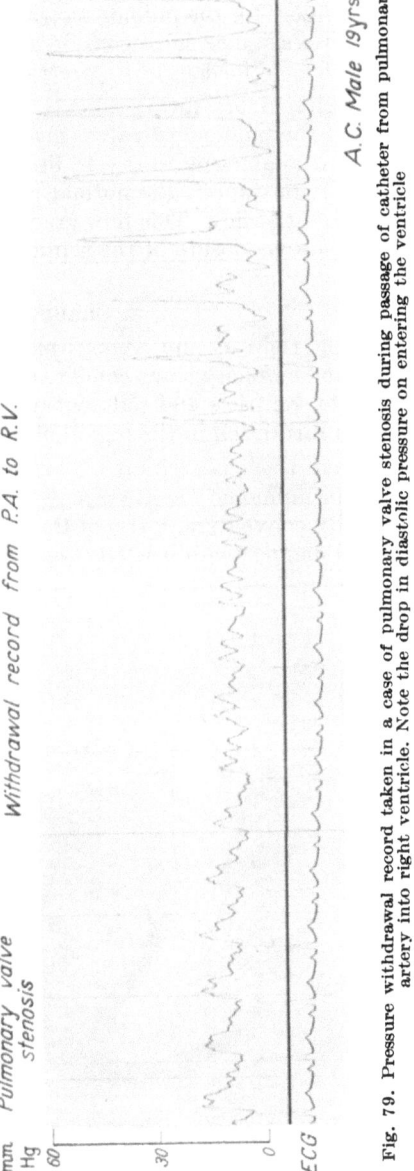

Fig. 79. Pressure withdrawal record taken in a case of pulmonary valve stenosis during passage of catheter from pulmonary artery into right ventricle. Note the drop in diastolic pressure on entering the ventricle

right heart catheterization gives no direct information of the pressure in the left ventricle.

Pressure measurements are also of help in diagnosing hypertension in the pulmonary arterial system and in assessing its severity. The pulmonary arterial pressure, taken in conjunction with the left atrial pressure and the cardiac output, gives a figure for the pulmonary vascular resistance. Estimation of the pulmonary vascular resistance is of considerable importance in assessing the suitability of septal defects for surgical correction.

Functional pressure gradients are common when large volumes of blood traverse the pulmonary valve ring. For example, in atrial septal defect there may be a flow amounting to say 18 litres/min. passing through the right heart and in these circumstances, the normal pulmonary valve ring acts as an obstruction to this torrential flow. This flow gradient — often in the region of 20—30 mm.Hg., disappears on closure of the septal defect.

2. Changes of Oxygen Saturation

In the right atrium, venous blood from the superior vena cava, inferior vena cava, and coronary sinus come together and the resultant mixture passes through the right ventricle and pulmonary vessels to the lungs. This blood has a venous oxygen saturation in the region of 65—75%.

Where there is a shunt of "arterial" blood into the right atrium, right ventricle, or pulmonary artery, there is a rise of oxygen saturation at the appropriate level. By convention, a rise of O_2 content of 2 vols.% in the right atrium is considered diagnostic of a left-to-right shunt at atrial level; while a rise of 1 vol.% and of $\frac{1}{2}$ vol.% at the right ventricular and pulmonary artery levels respectively, indicates a ventricular septal defect or aorto-pulmonary communication.

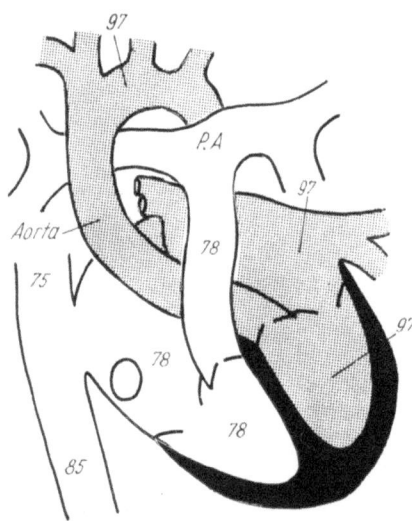

Fig. 80. Diagram indicating the approximate figures for the degree of oxygen saturation of the blood in the heart and great vessels

By estimating the degree of saturation of the blood in a systemic artery (by arterial needle puncture) it is possible to calculate separately the amount of blood flow through the pulmonary vascular bed and the systemic vascular bed. In this way one can calculate the volume of the shunt from one circulation to the other in litres per minute. Also, if the systemic arterial blood is desaturated, it is likely to indicate the presence of a right-to-left shunt of venous blood into the left side.

It should be borne in mind that the inferior caval blood may have a higher oxygen saturation than that in the superior vena cava due to the return of a stream of fairly highly saturated blood from the kidneys. The kidneys act as blood filters and the volume of blood passing through them is well in excess of their parenchymal oxygen requirements. Consequently, the returning blood in the renal veins may have a relatively high oxygen saturation.

On the other hand, the myocardium extracts a great deal of oxygen from the blood so that the coronary venous blood entering the right atrium from the coronary sinus has a lower oxygen saturation (about 40%) than any other blood in the body. If the cardiac catheter in the right atrium samples a stream of blood from the region of the coronary sinus, or if the catheter enters this orifice, the blood sample obtained will have a deceptively low oxygen saturation.

3. The Abnormal Passage of the Catheter

In following the passage of the catheter through the heart and out into the pulmonary arteries it may be seen to take an abnormal course and this observation can contribute information of diagnostic value. For example, the catheter may cross the atrial septum into the left atrium, confirming the presence of an atrial septal defect or a persistent foramen ovale. In ventricular septal defect the catheter may cross into the left ventricle or, more likely, pass out into the aorta, and in persistent ductus arteriosus the ductus is catheterized directly in about 70% of cases.

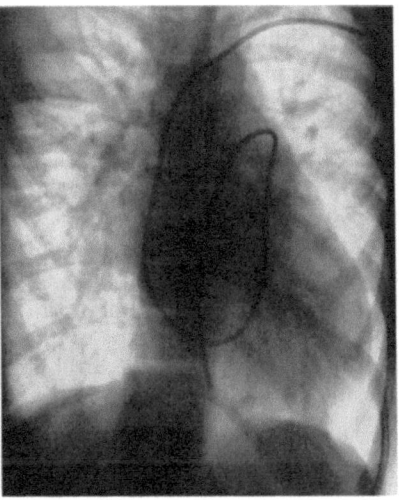

Again, the catheter may pass into a pulmonary vein from the venae cavae or from the right atrium and establish a diagnosis of anomalous pulmonary venous drainage or the course of the catheter may suggest transposition of the great vessels.

The information obtained at cardiac catheterization can be of great value in making a diagnosis, but it is subject to certain limitations. These may arise from errors in the technique of blood sampling and analysis or in the recording of pressure measurements. In addition, an incorrect interpretation may be placed on

Fig. 81. The cardiac catheter has passed through the right heart chambers, pulmonary artery and ductus to enter the descending aorta

the data received. Again, information is generally collected over a period of a few heart beats during the patient's life, and only reflects the pressures and oxygen saturation of the blood at that time and under conditions of the examination which might be quite abnormal. This applies particularly to an apprehensive patients at the end of a long and difficult catheterization.

A sound principle to adopt is that if the catheter results are totally at variance with the history and observed physical signs, radiography, and electrocardiography, the catheter results are probably wrong and should be disregarded or the investigation should be repeated.

Left Heart Catheterization

Right heart catheterization supplies information of pressure and oxygen saturation from all the cardiac chambers except the left ventricle; the left atrial pressure being derived from the pulmonary capillary samples (p. 61). By inserting an indwelling needle into the brachial artery it is also possible to obtain information about the circulation distal to the left ventricle. However, left ventricular pressures are unavailable. The measurement of the pressure in the left ventricle enables one to estimate the diastolic gradient across the mitral valve and the systolic pressure gradient across the aortic valve.

Information from the left heart chambers is obtainable in a number of ways.
  (1) Left atrial puncture
      (a) Bronchoscopic puncture
      (b) Percutaneous puncture through the back
      (c) Suprasternal puncture
  (2) Percutaneous left ventricular puncture.

1. Left Atrial Puncture

This technique was first described by ALLISON. He punctured the left atrium by means of a long needle passed under vision through a bronchoscope. The needle punctured the bronchial wall just lateral to the carina where the tracheal bifurcation straddles the left atrium.

By connecting the needle to an electromanometer, pressures can be recorded directly from the left atrium and this technique has been used to confirm the validity of pulmonary capillary wedge pressures as a measure of left atrial pressures.

The method has been developed further so that a long fine catheter can be passed down the needle and through the mitral valve into the left ventricle. In this way, left atrial and left ventricular pressures can be recorded synchronously and are of value in assessing mitral valve disease.

An alternative approach to the left atrium was introduced by BJORK, of Sweden. He described percutaneous needle puncture of the left atrium from the back; the needle entering about the level of the 9th rib in the right paravertebral area and passing medially beyond the vertebral body.

The patient lies either on his left side or, more conveniently, on his face and a thin catheter can be passed through the needle into the left atrium and manipulated into the left ventricle during continuous pressure observations. This method is quite frequently used in difficult cases of mitral valve disease. The investigation is associated with a fair incidence of pain, stiffness and morbidity.

An alternative route is to pass a fine needle through the skin in the suprasternal notch or supraclavicular fossa, down through the aorta, measuring this pressure en route, and also possibly through the pulmonary artery before entering the left atrium.

2. Left Ventricular Puncture

Where one is dealing with aortic valve disease it is of great help to be able to record the left ventricular pressure directly. This can be accomplished safely and simply by percutaneous needle puncture of the left ventricle at the point where the hypertrophied left ventricle impinges against the chest wall. Also at the apex of the heart there are no large coronary arteries to be damaged.

The procedure can be rapidly carried out and is well tolerated under local infiltration analgesia. A simultaneous pressure recorded from the brachial artery gives a measure of the systolic pressure drop over the aortic valve, but this information can be obtained more exactly by passing a fine catheter through the left ventricular needle and aortic valve into the aorta. On withdrawing this catheter slowly, one obtains not only information about the pressure gradient but also about the site of stenosis. In this way it is possible to make a precise distinction between valve stenosis and subvalvar aortic stenosis. In addition supravalvar stenosis can be diagnosed by this method.

If measurements of the cardiac output are made at the time, one can calculate the approximate size of the aortic valve orifice.

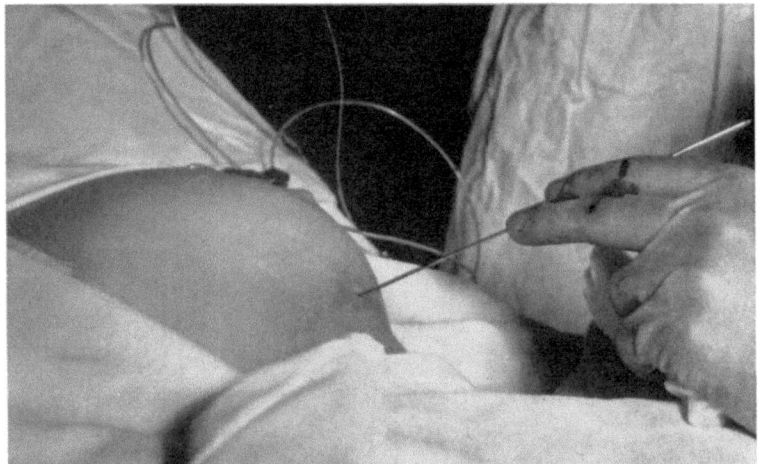

Fig. 82. Left ventricular puncture. The needle is inserted into the left ventricle at the point at which the impulse is clearly felt. Pressures are recorded by means of an electromanometer

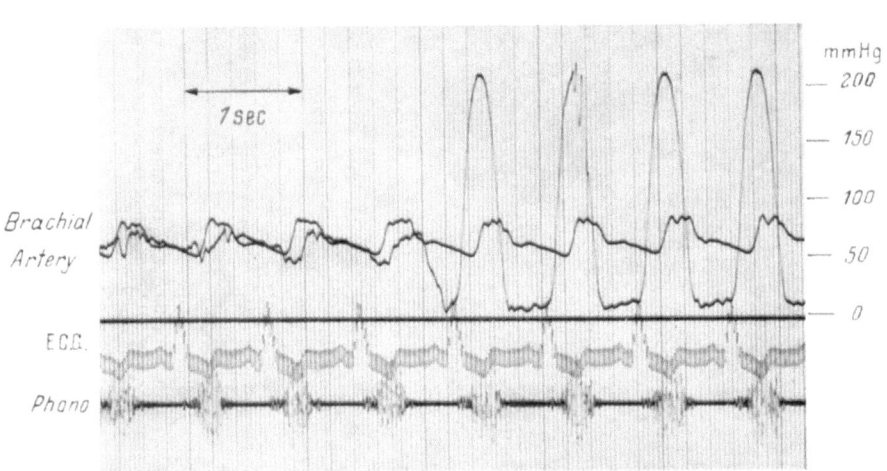

Fig. 83a. As the catheter passes from aorta to left ventricle, there is the normal drop of diastolic pressure as the valve is passed but also a systolic gradient, amounting to about 120 mm., becomes apparent. The simultaneous brachial artery trace overlies the aortic and left ventricular records

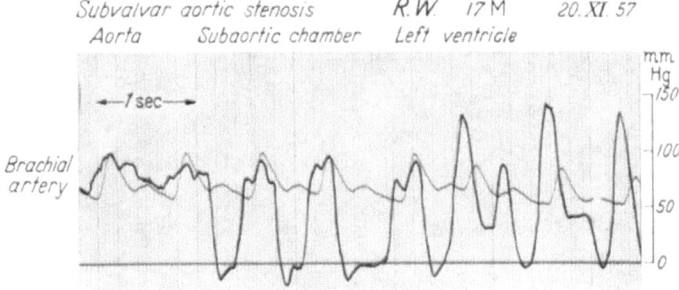

Fig. 83b. In this case of subvalvar aortic stenosis, the passage across the valve is indicated by the **fall** of diastolic pressure but the systolic gradient only appears at a lower level. Faint line indicates **brachial** artery pressure

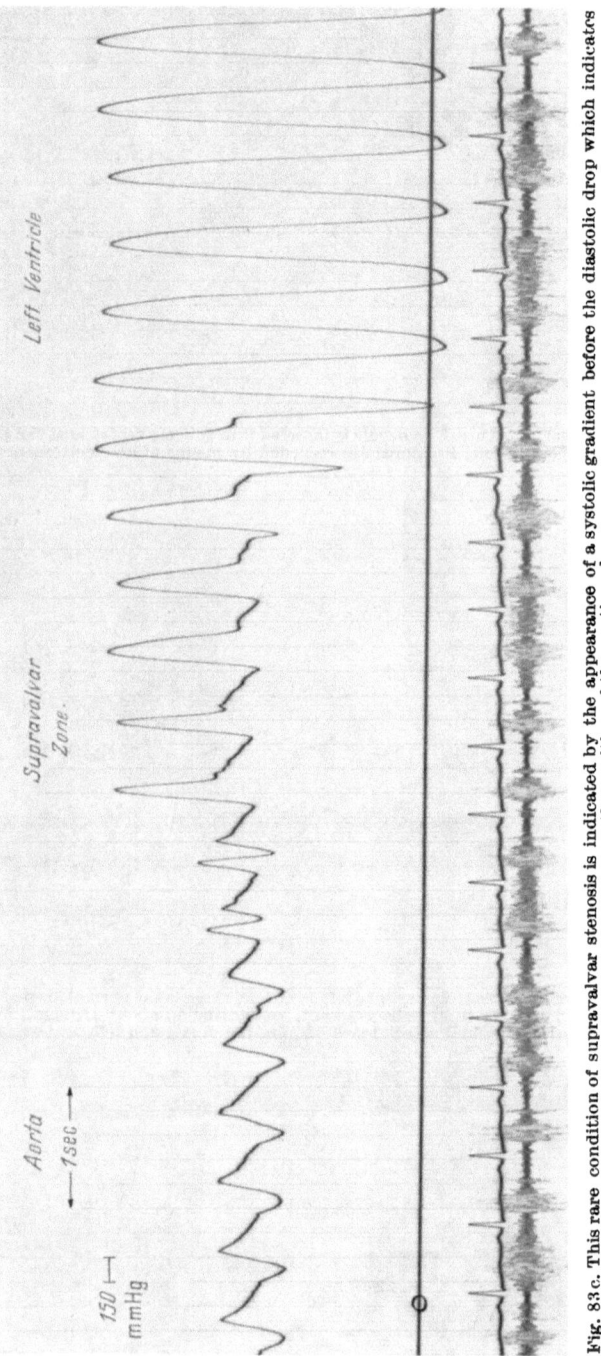

Fig. 83c. This rare condition of supravalvar stenosis is indicated by the appearance of a systolic gradient before the diastolic drop which indicates the position of the aortic valve

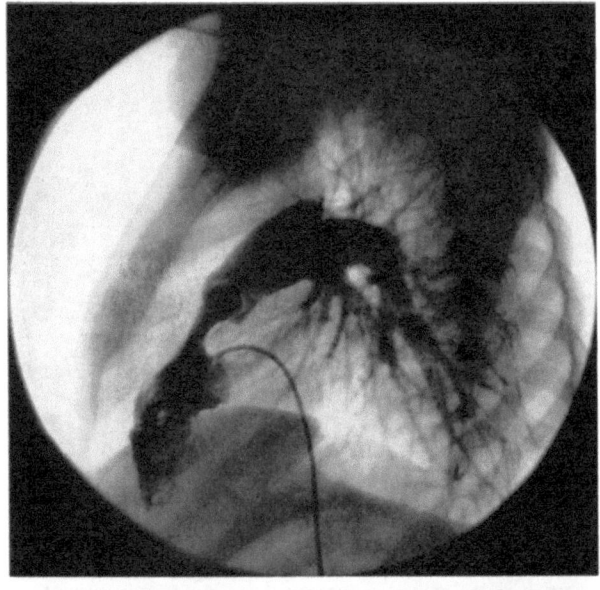

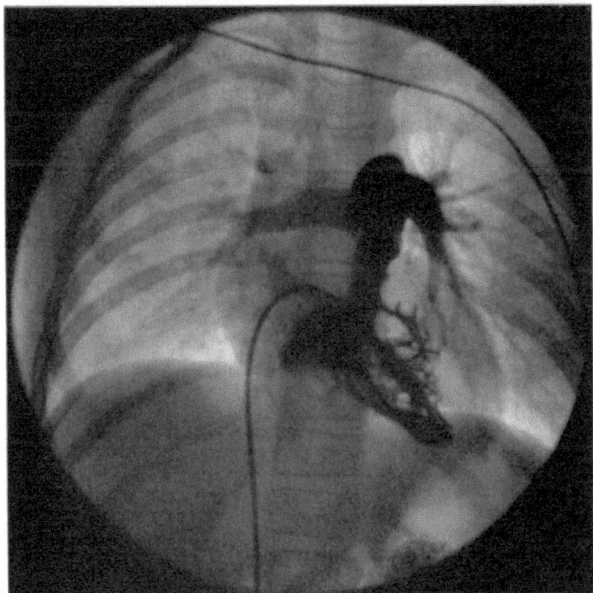

Fig. 84a and b. An angiocardiogram obtained by injecting contrast medium directly into the right ventricle. The infundibulum and valve are clearly demonstrated

Angiocardiography

This is a technique for visualising the cardiac chambers and associated great vessels by means of injected contrast medium. The resulting X-ray shadows are recorded with a high-speed exposure of up to six to twelve frames per second.

As a rule, an injection of 70—90% iodine compound is made into a cannula in one of the arm veins or via a catheter passed directly into the right atrium or right ventricle. About 1.5 ml./per kg. is injected — the dosage varying from 0.75 mg. to 2 ml/per kg. Where selective visualisation of, say, the right ventricular outflow

5*

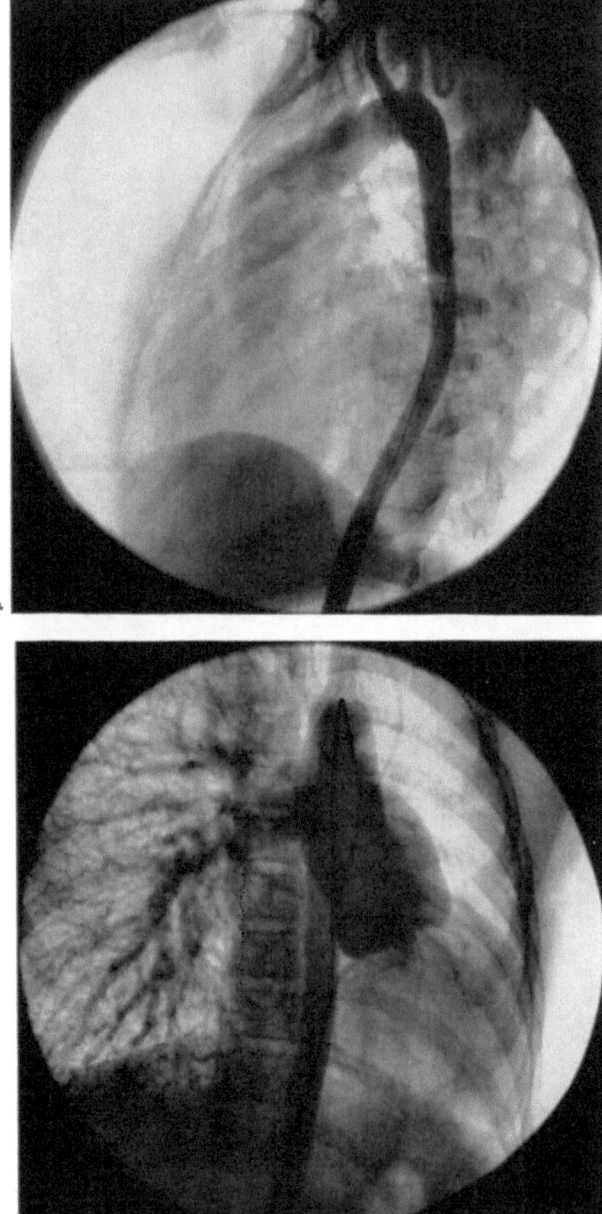

Fig. 85a and b. Retrograde aortograms. The lateral aortogram has been used to exclude the presence of a persistent ductus arteriosus. The postero-anterior projection demonstrated an aorto-pulmonary window defect

is required, it is usual to position the catheter in the right ventricle and to inject smaller amounts of contrast medium.

The examination is performed under general anaesthetic in children but in adults sedation only may be used, although there may be unpleasant but transient symptoms.

Angiocardiography is chiefly of value in conditions associated with a right-to-left shunt, as in FALLOT's tetralogy, since the contrast medium is carried across from the right heart to the left with the shunt stream.

Considerable effort is being directed towards improving the detail and information available and among the available techniques, cine-angiocardiography has established a place. In this technique, contrast medium is again injected but the X-ray picture is projected on an image intensifier which is photographed by a ciné-camera. The film, when projected, not only indicates the passage of the blood, but gives information of the functional activity of the various heart chambers and of the degree of shunt.

Another development is to project the image on an image intensifier, which is then visualised by a television camera, so that the procedure can be monitored on a number of screens and recorded on film. These techniques, using image intensification and ciné-camera or television screening, reduce the exposure of the operator and patient to radiation.

Aortography

This is allied to arteriography, and is used to visualise the aorta and limb arteries. Lumbar aortography is performed by injection through a needle passed into the abdominal aorta from the back. The needle is usually inserted just above

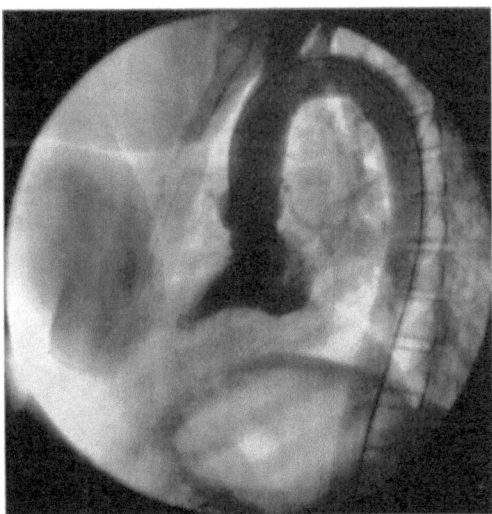 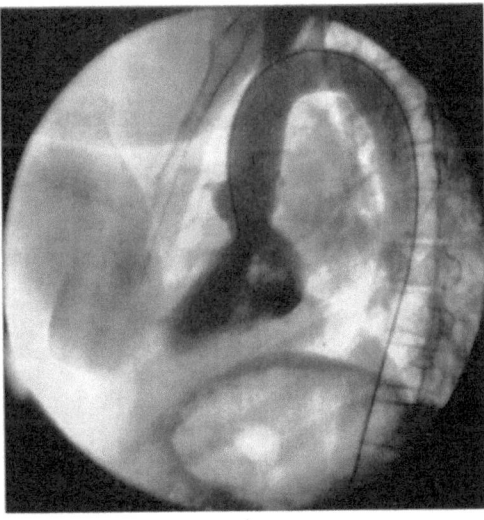

a   b

Fig. 86. Left ventricular angiograms in a case of mitral valve disease. The pictures coincide with systole (a) and diastole (b) and show negligible regurgitation

the renal arteries. Alternatively, the femoral artery is punctured and a catheter is threaded through this into the abdominal aorta.

Retrograde aortography can be of considerable value in demonstrating persistent ductus arteriosus and in differentiating this condition from ventricular septal defect where the evidence obtained at catheterization is inconclusive. The injection is usually made into the ascending aorta via a catheter passed up from the brachial or femoral artery and guided into position with the aid of fluoroscopy. Not only can a ductus be demonstrated, but also a deformed or regurgitant aortic valve can be visualised and, in some cases, the coronary arteries are also outlined.

Coronary angiography is a development of retrograde aortography. In order to obtain a good visualisation of the coronary vessels it may be necessary to inject acetylcholine or a related drug to produce extreme bradycardia. Alternatively the vessels can be intubated with a fine catheter.

Left ventricular angiography, in which contrast medium is injected directly into the left ventricle by percutaneous puncture or by retrograde passage of an aortic catheter enables one to demonstrate left-to-right shunts through a ventricular septal defect and also regurgitation at the mitral valve.

Selected List of References for Further Reading

Auscultation of the Heart. Aubrey Leatham. Goulstonian Lecture (1958) Lancet 2, 703.

The Anatomy of Congenital Pulmonary Stenosis. R. C. Brock. (1957) Cassell & Co. Ltd, London.

Functional Obstruction of the Left Ventricle. R. C. Brock (1957) Guy's Hosp. Rep. 106, 221.

The Eisenmenger Syndrome or Pulmonary Hypertension with Reversed Central Shunt. Paul Wood. Croonian Lecture. (1958) Brit. med. J. 2, 701.

The Obscure Physiology of Poststenotic Dilitation: Its Relation to the Development of Aneurysms. Holman, E. (1954) J. thorac. Surg. 28, 109.

Index